Fundamentals of Nuclear Medicine

Fundamentals of Nuclear Medicine

Second Edition

EDITORS

Naomi P. Alazraki, M.D.
Co-Director, Nuclear Medicine
and Professor of Radiology
Emory University School of Medicine
Atlanta, Georgia

Fred S. Mishkin, M.D.
Nuclear Medicine Section
Memorial Medical Center of Long Beach
and Clinical Professor of Radiology
UCLA School of Medicine
Los Angeles, California

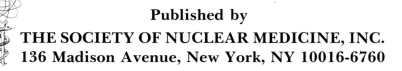

Published by
THE SOCIETY OF NUCLEAR MEDICINE, INC.
136 Madison Avenue, New York, NY 10016-6760

The Society of Nuclear Medicine, Inc.
136 Madison Ave. New York, NY 10016-6760

First edition published in 1984.

Made in the United States of America

Library of Congress Cataloging in Publication Data

Fundamentals of nuclear medicine. / editors, Naomi P. Alazraki, Fred S. Mishkin.—2nd ed.
    p.   cm.
   Includes bibliographies and index.
   ISBN 0-932004-29-6
   1. Radioisotope scanning. 2. Nuclear medicine. I. Alazraki, Naomi P. II. Mishkin, Fred S., 1937-
   [DNLM: 1. Nuclear Medicine.   WN 440 F981]
RC78.7.R4F83 1988
616.07'575—dc19
DNLM/DLC
for Library of Congress   88-4658
                                            CIP

Printing: 2 3 4 5 6 7 8   Year: 8 9 0

Preface to Second Edition

The widespread acceptance of this small volume to help introduce fundamental nuclear medicine principles to medical students has prompted this update. In a continually changing diagnostic field, currency and perspective without bulk pose a difficult challenge. We have tried to present a balanced approach to the diagnostic value of nuclear medicine procedures, emphasizing what they do best, as well as pointing out their limitations. The exciting promise of positron emission tomography, which is providing unique insights into body chemistry and function, is outlined in this update. Our intent is to provide an introduction to this rapidly evolving technology as it emerges from the investigative into the clinical stage.

We appreciate the cooperation of all contributors and many others without whose contributed efforts this work could not have been completed in a timely fashion. We would especially like to acknowledge the efforts of Richard Witcofski, Ph.D., Chairman of the Publications Committee, and William D. Kaplan, M.D., Chairman of the Education and Training Committee of the Society of Nuclear Medicine. We are indebted to those in the Central Office of the Society of Nuclear Medicine, particularly David Teisler, Toni Ann Scaramuzzo, and Eleanore Tapscott, whose patience and generous help brought forth this new edition with a minimum of delay and aggravation.

The Editors

Preface to First Edition

This basic guidebook for clinical nuclear medicine is written as an easily readable description of how nuclear medicine procedures should be used by clinicians in evaluating their patients. It is designed to assist medical students and physicians in becoming acquainted with the major useful nuclear medicine techniques for detecting and evaluating common disorders. The material provides an introduction to, not a textbook of, nuclear medicine; it has been written in a manner that will encourage a medical student or physician to read it in an evening or two.

Each chapter is devoted to a particular organ system or topic relevant to an understanding and appreciation of the risks and benefits involved in nuclear medicine studies. The basics of radiation and evaluation of radiation risk in the perspective of the levels of natural environmental radiation are presented to educate physicians. The awareness and sensitivities of the general public toward the topic of radiation demand that all clinicians who refer patients for studies using ionizing radiation have a basic understanding of radiation. Chapter 1 places the phenomenon of radiation in perspective.

The emphasis is on presenting the rationales for ordering the various clinical imaging procedures performed in most nuclear medicine departments. An Appendix summarizes the approximate sensitivities and specificities of various radionuclide studies for particular diseases or physiologic evaluations. The sensitivities and specificities listed represent the consensus of estimations submitted by a group of knowledgeable practicing nuclear medicine physicians. Selected Readings are listed at the end of each chapter for those interested in obtaining additional information.

A glossary of nomenclature and terms used in discussions of nuclear medicine and radiation is included. In addition to the clinical emphasis of this manual, a brief explanation of how the imaging equipment works is provided. Discussion of nonimaging studies, including the in vitro radioimmunoassay procedures, is included.

Although the chapters are primarily organized according to organ systems, some chapters deal with specific categories of problems or diseases; for example, Chapters 11–13 are devoted to evaluation of trauma, infectious or inflammatory lesions, and cancer. Where appropriate, alternative imaging modalities including ultrasound, computed tomography imaging, and radiographic special procedures are discussed. Comparative data between nuclear medicine imaging and other modalities are presented to help guide the practicing clinician in the selection of the most appropriate procedure for a given problem. Clinical experience with nuclear magnetic resonance as an imaging modality is not yet sufficiently established at the time of this writing to permit comparative data relative to radionuclide studies.

The editors wish to acknowledge and express thanks for valuable guidance and help from James A. Sorenson, Ph.D., Book Coordinator of the Society of Nuclear Medicine, from C. Douglas Maynard, M.D., Chairman of the Publications Committee, and from Peter Kirchner, M.D., who was Chairman of the Education and Training Committee during the development of this document. We are grateful to Ms. Laura Kosden, Ms. Karen Schools, and Ms. Laura Schraub of the Central Office of the Society of Nuclear Medicine for their valuable advice, help, and support for this publication.

The Editors

Contents

RADIATION IN PERSPECTIVE

1. **Basic Science of Nuclear Medicine** *3*
   Radiation and Dose *3*
   Radiation Effects *6*
   Radiopharmaceuticals *11*
   Imaging of Radiation *15*
   Positron Emission Tomography *16*
   Single-Photon Emission Computed
      Tomography *18*
   Selected Readings *19*

2. **The Diagnostic Process and Nuclear
   Medicine** *21*
   Sensitivity, Specificity, and Receiver Operating
      Characteristic Curve *22*
   Predictive Value, Prevalence, and Bayes'
      Theorem *24*
   Selected Readings *30*

ORGAN IMAGING WITH RADIONUCLIDES

3. **Endocrinology** *35*
   Thyroid Uptake and Imaging *35*
   Radioiodine Therapy *42*
   Thyroid Carcinoma *43*
   Parathyroid Imaging *44*
   Adrenal Cortical Uptake and Imaging *47*
   Adrenal Medullary Imaging *49*
   Selected Readings *51*

4. **Cardiovascular System** *53*
   Cardiac Blood-Pool Imaging and Evaluation of
      Ventricular Function *53*
   Radionuclide Angiocardiography *58*
   Evaluation of Myocardial Perfusion *59*

PET Imaging, Blood Flow, and Metabolism   *63*
Myocardial Infarct Imaging   *64*
Selected Readings   *66*

5. **Pulmonary System and Thromboembolism**   *68*
Diagnosis of Pulmonary Embolism   *68*
Principles of Pulmonary Perfusion/Ventilation
   Imaging   *69*
Ventilation Imaging   *70*
Sensitivity of Pulmonary Perfusion Imaging in
   Detecting Pulmonary Embolism   *71*
Specificity of Radionuclide Pulmonary Perfusion
   Imaging   *71*
Nonembolic Pulmonary Disease   *76*
Thrombus Detection   *76*
Selected Readings   *81*

6. **Liver and Gastrointestinal Tract**   *83*
Liver–Spleen Imaging   *83*
Esophagus, Stomach, and Duodenum   *87*
Acute Gastrointestinal Hemorrhage   *91*
Selected Readings   *92*

7. **Biliary Tract**   *95*
Cholecystitis   *95*
Biliary Leakage   *99*
Cholestasis   *99*
Postoperative Evaluation   *99*
Trauma   *100*
Selected Readings   *100*

8. **Genitourinary Tract**   *102*
Evaluation of Renal Function   *103*
Hydronephrosis or Possible Obstruction   *105*
Ureteral Reflux   *108*
Renal Parenchymal Masses   *108*
Renovascular Hypertension   *109*
Renal Transplantation   *109*
Scrotal Imaging (Torsion versus Epididymitis)   *110*
Selected Readings   *110*

9. Skeletal System *112*

Principles of Radionuclide Bone Imaging *112*

Neoplasms *113*

Trauma *116*

Vascular Disease *117*

Infection *117*

Metabolic Disease *118*

Joint Disease *118*

Soft Tissue Lesions *120*

Selected Readings *120*

10. Central Nervous System *123*

PET Imaging *123*

SPECT Imaging *126*

Radionuclide Cerebral Angiography *127*

Delayed Brain Scan Images *130*

Cerebrospinal Fluid Dynamics *132*

Selected Readings *135*

IMAGING DISEASE PROCESSES

11. Trauma *139*

Brain *139*

Liver *140*

Spleen *140*

Kidney *141*

Vascular *142*

Bone *142*

Lung *145*

Selected Readings *145*

12. Inflammatory and Infectious Processes *148*

Multiorgan Imaging *148*

Gallium-67 Imaging *150*

Indium-111-Labeled Leukocytes *153*

Selected Readings *155*

13. Cancer *157*

Radionuclide Liver Imaging *157*

Radionuclide Lymphoscintigraphy *159*

Evaluation of the Chest   *161*
Radioimmunodetection and Radioimmunotherapy   *164*
Specific Tumor Types   *167*
Selected Readings   *170*

NONIMAGING DIAGNOSTIC TECHNIQUES

14. **Nonimaging Procedures**   *175*
Radioligand Assays   *175*
Schilling Test   *178*
Measuring Body Spaces   *180*
Other Nonimaging Quantitative Tests   *184*
Selected Readings   *187*

Appendix   *189*

Glossary   *203*

Index   *226*

Contributors

Naomi P. Alazraki, M.D.
Co-Director, Nuclear Medicine
Professor of Radiology
Emory University School of
  Medicine
Atlanta, Georgia

Fredrick L. Datz, M.D.
Director, Nuclear Medicine
The University of Utah Medical
  Center;
Associate Professor of Radiology
The University of Utah Medical
  School
Salt Lake City, Utah

William D. Kaplan, M.D.
Associate Professor of Radiology
Harvard Medical School
Chief, Oncologic Nuclear
  Medicine
Dana Farber Cancer Institute
Boston, Massachusetts

Lorna K. Mee, Ph.D.
Principal Research Associate in
  Radiology (Nuclear Medicine)
Shields Warren Radiation
  Laboratory
Harvard Medical School
Boston, Massachusetts

Fred S. Mishkin, M.D.
Nuclear Medicine Section
Memorial Medical Center of
  Long Beach
Clinical Professor of Radiology
UCLA School of Medicine
Los Angeles, California

Dennis D. Patton, M.D.
Professor of Radiology
Director of the Division of
  Nuclear Medicine
Arizona Health Sciences Center
Tucson, Arizona

Isaac C. Reese, Ph.D.
Department of Radiology
King/Drew Medical Center;
Professor of Radiology
Charles R. Drew University of
  Medicine and Science
Los Angeles, California

Barry A. Siegel, M.D.
Director, Division of Nuclear
  Medicine,
Mallinckrodt Institute of
  Radiology;
Professor of Radiology and
  Medicine,
Washington University School
  of Medicine
St. Louis, Missouri

James A. Sorenson, Ph.D.
Director, Research
Lunar Corporation
Madison, Wisconsin

Andrew T. Taylor, Jr., M.D.
Co-Director, Nuclear Medicine
Professor of Radiology
Emory University School of
  Medicine
Atlanta, Georgia

Heidi S. Weissmann, M.D.
Formerly,
Associate Professor of Nuclear
    Medicine and Radiology
Albert Einstein College of
    Medicine
Bronx, New York

Henry N. Wellman, M.D.
Director, Nuclear Medicine
    Division,
Indiana University Hospital;
Professor of Medicine and
    Radiology
Indiana University Medical
    Center
Indianapolis, Indiana

James M. Woolfenden, M.D.
Professor of Radiology
Division of Nuclear Medicine
Arizona Health Sciences Center
Tucson, Arizona

Contributors to First Edition

Manuel L. Brown, M.D.
Mayo Clinic
Rochester, Minnesota

Leon S. Malmud, M.D.
Temple University
Philadelphia, Pennsylvania

Leroy A. Sugarman, M.D.
Albert Einstein College of
    Medicine
Bronx, New York

Radiation in Perspective

1

Basic Science of Nuclear Medicine

RADIATION AND DOSE

Energy emitted by atoms undergoing internal change, transferred through space or matter, is called radiation. Medical diagnostic imaging has used chiefly *ionizing* radiation in the form of x-rays and γ-rays. β-particles and α-particles, also forms of ionizing radiation, may contribute to radiation dose in medical procedures, but are not useful for imaging, mainly because they travel distances of only a few millimeters in tissue. In addition to ionizing radiation, nonionizing radiation in the lower-energy portion of the electromagnetic spectrum, radiofrequency (RF), is used in the process of magnetic resonance imaging (MRI) to induce changes in the nuclei of atoms that have been placed in a stable, uniformly graded magnetic field. Images are formed from the recorded tissue responses to the RF signal in the magnetic field. Medical imaging also employs ultrasound (coherent, high-frequency sound wave radiation) to form images by reflection from tissue interfaces of different acoustic impedances. This chapter deals with ionizing radiation and its effects on human beings.

The amount of radiation energy absorbed by irradiated tissue is called radiation dose and is specified in grays (1 Gy = 100 rad)* or in rads or millirads (1/1000 rad).* A dose of 1 rad

---

*Throughout this book we use both traditional radiation units: rads, rems, roentgens, curies, and SI (Système Internationale) units. Students and practitioners are encouraged to become familiar with SI units (see Appendix).

3

implies 100 erg of energy absorbed per gram of tissue and 1 gray implies 1 joule of energy per kilogram of tissue. A closely related quantity, called dose equivalent, relates the dose to biologic risk and is specified in sieverts (1 Sv = 100 rem) or rems. For practical purposes, a dose of 0.01 Gy or 1 rad from x-rays or radiation associated with nuclear medical procedures delivers a dose equivalent of 0.01 Sv or 1 rem. Some types of radiation associated with nuclear weapons (e.g., α-particles and neutrons) have greater potential for biologic damage and deliver dose equivalents of 10–20 Sv/Gy or 10–20 rem/rad of dose. Finally, the quantity exposure refers to the amount of ionization produced by a beam of x-rays or γ-rays in air and is used to specify radiation levels in the environment. The basic unit is the roentgen (R). Exposure levels are measured with radiation detection devices such as ionization chambers and Geiger counters. For x-rays and γ-rays, when the measured exposure level is 1 R, the dose that would be delivered to a mass of tissue located at that same point would be ~0.01 Gy or 1 rad. For radiation used for medical diagnostic purposes, roentgens, rads, and rems turn out to be numerically equivalent, although they actually represent different quantities.

The major difference between electromagnetic radiation, such as x-rays and γ-rays, and particulate radiation, such as β-particles and α-particles, lies in their ability to penetrate matter. Whereas β-particles travel only a few millimeters and α-particles travel less than 100 μm in soft tissue before expending all their energy, x-rays and γ-rays distribute their energy more diffusely and can traverse many centimeters of tissue. Hence, β-particles and α-particles deliver highly localized radiation doses, whereas x-rays and γ-rays deliver doses more uniformly throughout the irradiated tissues. The dose concentration of β-particles is used to advantage, for example, in the treatment of hyperthyroidism with radioiodine, because the selective uptake of iodine by the thyroid gland results in highly selective irradiation of that organ. In contrast, for external-beam therapy, x-rays or γ-rays from linear accelerators or cobalt-60 machines are used to treat larger volumes of tissue to a more uniform dose level. For a given dose level and dose distribution, however, x-, γ-, and β-radiation have similar biologic and therapeutic effects.

Although significant gaps in our knowledge persist, we have learned a great deal about the deleterious effects associated with tissue radiation. We know that a sharp and decisive distinction must be made between the acute and subacute effects produced by massive amounts of radiation, for example, from nuclear bombs or radiation for cancer therapy, and those long-term effects produced by the low levels of medical radiation for diagnosis, which differ in dose levels by factors of thousands or more. An understanding of natural environmental radiation, which also constitutes a source of low-level radiation exposure, is useful in placing medical radiation in proper perspective.

Background Radiation

Radiation from cosmic rays and from naturally occurring radioactive atoms results in variable background irradiation, depending on where we live. Major differences exist between sea level and high altitudes and between regions of different soil and rock compositions. In Florida, for example, the average annual background radiation approximates 0.8–1.0 mSv (80–100 mrem)/year, whereas in some high regions of India, exposures measure up to 13 mSv (1300 mrem)/year. Background radiation in the Denver–Boulder, Colorado area is twice that at sea level. If one lives in a brick building, the naturally occurring radioactivity in the material used to make the brick increases background irradiation above that of a wood building. Perhaps the greatest variability in background radiation is due to indoor radon, which exposes the bronchial epithelium to α-particle irradiation.

The human body contains natural radioactivity as well. Approximately 0.01% of our body potassium is radioactive potassium-40 (3.7 kBq; 1 Bq = 27 picocuries ~0.1 μCi).* Our bodies also contain about the same amount of carbon-14. Currently, laboratory animals containing this amount of injected radioactivity are considered radioactive, yet no one considers the normal human body radioactive. In the United States, natural radiation

---

*The Becquerel (Bq) and Curie (Ci) are units of radioactivity (see Appendix).

results in an estimated average annual dose equivalent of about 1.4 mSv (140 mrem).

The chief source of increased radiation to human beings over background levels is medical diagnostic radiation. Although such levels are not delivered uniformly to the entire population, calculations made as if they were suggest that this source contributes an average of 1.53–3 mSv (153–300 mrem) per person per year in the United States. Dental examinations and radiation exposure in certain occupations contribute additional increased radiation doses. Radioactive lead-210 and polonium-210 have been observed in cigarette smoke and in the bronchial epithelium of cigarette smokers. Modern air travel increases the exposure of the public to radiation. At 30,000 ft, passengers on polar flights receive an additional 0.01 mSv (1 mrem)/hr, while mid-latitude flights yield exposures of 5 μSv (0.5 mrem)/hr.

RADIATION EFFECTS

Risks from Radiation

Radiation effects on human beings may be classified as *somatic*, affecting the irradiated person, or *genetic*, affecting progeny. Delayed somatic effects include cancer. The ability to predict whether a certain level of radiation will be harmful to a given person or to an entire population hinges on the probability of radiation effect that is dose dependent and assumed to be without a threshold value. Thus, in the absence of a threshold, a very small dose would result in a small increase in the probability that a certain radiation effect will occur. At the level of radiation from diagnostic studies, the increase over background is so small that increases in effects (e.g., cancer) over those that occur naturally in the general population are difficult if not impossible to demonstrate by epidemiologic methods.

High-Level Radiation Doses and Somatic Effects

Early somatic changes occur after relatively large doses of radiation. These are the changes associated in the popular mind with radiation: hair loss, skin burns, loss of oral and intestinal mucosal integrity, failure of production of short-lived cells, aspermia, agranulocytosis, sepsis, generalized debility, and death.

The eventual survival time and mode of death after whole body exposure depend on the dose level. At very high doses of 100–150 Gy (10,000–15,000 rad), death occurs in a few hours and appears to result from neurologic and cardiovascular breakdown—central nervous system (CNS) syndrome. At dose levels of 5–12 Gy (500–1200 rad), death occurs within a few days and results from destruction of the gastrointestinal (GI) mucosa (GI syndrome). At lower dose levels of 2.5–5.0 Gy (250–500 rad), death occurs several weeks after exposure, due to effects on bone marrow (hematopoietic syndrome). The exact cause of death in the CNS syndrome is unclear. In the GI and hematopoietic syndromes, the principal cause of death is the depletion of the stem cells of the epithelium of the gut or of the circulating blood cells. The difference in the dose level and time at which these two forms of death occur reflects variations in the population kinetics of the two cell-renewal systems, and differences in the amount of damage that can be tolerated. In addition to standard medical therapy, treatment for the hematopoietic syndrome has included extensive bone marrow transplants, as was performed in the individuals exposed in the nuclear accident at Chernobyl.

Somatic changes do result from, and are actually the purpose of, therapeutic irradiation. For example, reduced thyroid function is the aim of treating hyperthyroidism with radioactive iodine (^{131}I). Sialitis may occur as an undesirable somatic side effect. Hypothyroidism, a somatic change, is a frequently occurring result. Chromosomal changes can be found after such treatment, but long-term follow-up of many such treated patients who have had children shows no increased incidence of either genetic damage or carcinogenesis. Although the incidence of leukemia is increased over that seen in the general population, it is not more than that of the population with hyperthyroidism treated by surgery without radiation. Therapeutic doses of irradiation, for example, those delivered by radioiodide for the treatment of thyroid cancer, are approximately 10–12 times higher than doses delivered for benign disease. Such doses are associated with more long-lived chromosomal damage.

Somatic changes usually associated with multiple doses of radioactivity used in high-level cancer therapy include bone marrow depression, enteritis, and tissue or organ fibrosis if there is undue concentration of the radioactivity in a particular organ.

Radiation Carcinogenesis

Since the earliest use of x-rays, radiation production of tumors has been noted. Carcinogenesis has been postulated to require an initiator and a promoter. The usually long latent period—decades—between radiation exposure and the appearance of a tumor suggests radiation does not create malignant cells per se, but functions as an initiator.

Radiation-induced cancer has been observed in several populations: lung cancer in uranium miners from the effects of inhalation of radon on the lung epithelium, bone tumors in radium dial painters, and liver cancer in patients receiving Thorotrast®, a radioactive contrast agent. An unfortunate example of radiation-related cancer is the increase in thyroid cancer associated with thymic irradiation of approximately 1 Gy (100 rad) in infancy. This practice was performed 30–40 years ago to shrink an enlarged thymus. Even lower doses directed to the face to treat acne or to the scalp for ringworm produced an apparent increased incidence of thyroid cancer in children who had years previously received as little as 0.06–0.07 Gy (6–7 rad).

The most extensive data that permit a quantitative assessment of risk from radiation as a function of dose comes from the Japanese survivors of Hiroshima and Nagasaki and from the therapeutic exposure of patients with ankylosing spondylitis. A significant increase in the incidence of leukemia was found in the Japanese survivors, which peaked at ~10 yr after exposure and then declined. An elevated incidence of other cancers, including lung, breast, and thyroid cancers, has been detected; these cancers appear to have a longer latent period than leukemia. In spondylitic patients, an increased incidence of leukemia was found, which was comparable to that seen in the Japanese study.

The estimated risk for radiation-induced malignancy is based on these limited data using doses of 1 Gy (100 rad) or higher. Scientists have assumed that the mathematical relationship between dose and effect, linear, quadratic or linear quadratic, observed at high doses can be extrapolated back to low doses. If there is a threshold effect, or if the relationship is curvilinear, low doses could have considerably lower risk than predicted by this extrapolated risk estimate.*

Perhaps the major difficulty in estimating the incidence of cancer induced by low-level radiation is that the naturally occurring incidence of cancer is relatively high compared with any slight increase that might be expected from low doses of radiation. Studies have been reported linking radiation exposure in utero from pelvimetry and other x-ray studies with an increased incidence of childhood leukemia. The doubling dose, the dose required to double the "natural risk" (0.1%), suggested from these studies is a few millisieverts (rems). However, to date, no other studies have reliably shown an increase in cancer incidence at diagnostic radiation dose levels. Other studies, such as those of a population in Sweden that received diagnostic doses of ^{131}I, have specifically shown no increased incidence of thyroid cancer. Thus the risk of cancer from low-dose levels remains hypothetical according to extrapolations from data for persons exposed to higher-dose levels.

Genetic Effects

The descendants of the Japanese survivors of Hiroshima and Nagasaki are the largest population available for estimating the genetic hazards of radiation exposure. No increase has been observed in the incidence of prenatal or neonatal deaths or the frequency of malformations. However, the number of people

---

*A linear effect is $E = aD$. A linear quadratic effect is $E = aD + bD^2$, where E = radiation effect, and a and b are constants, and D = radiation dose.

exposed was small by genetic standards, and insufficient time has passed for the appearance of recessive mutations which require several generations for their expression.

The genetically significant dose (GSD) is useful in estimating the potential genetic impact from irradiation of large populations. It is calculated from a knowledge of the amount of radiation received by a given number of people, with a weighting factor applied to allow for the potential reproductive activity of the particular population. The GSD is the dose that, if received by all members of the population, would produce the same genetic effect as the doses which are in fact received by selected individuals within the population. The annual GSD from natural radiation is estimated to have an average value of 1.4 mSv (0.14 rem). Other than radon, diagnostic x-ray radiography contributes the largest source of additional radiation exposure to the U.S. population with an estimated annual GSD of 0.25 mSv (25 mrems). The GSD from nuclear medical procedures is estimated to be 0.02 mSv (2 mrems).

From these data regarding carcinogenic and genetic effects, incomplete as they are, the National Council of Radiation Protection (NCRP) has issued permissible dose standards for those who work with radiation [currently 0.05 Sv (5 rem)/year for total-body radiation doses].

For the general public, a suggested maximum annual permissible total body dose is in the mid-range of background radiation, about 5 mGy (500 mrad). No guides have been issued for patients; however, as a general rule, diagnostic testing should be conducted with the smallest radiation dose practical and the most favorable risk–benefit techniques available. Radiation, like any other agent with even low-level toxic potential, should be used only when indicated for diagnostic purposes. Particularly in patients who may be pregnant, or in children, physicians must have clearly good indications if radiation is used. In contrast, when a procedure that delivers ionizing radiation can yield information essential to the management of a patient, there should be no hesitation in using radiation. Therefore, when indicated, don't hesitate to use diagnostic radiation, but refrain from using radiation on a routine basis unless the benefit is established.

In the case of potentially pregnant women, special consideration should be given to the relatively high radiosensitivity of the fetus, particularly during the first trimester. Thus, it is important to ask when the patient had her last menstrual period and whether she suspects that she may be pregnant. If she responds that she could be pregnant, the procedure should be postponed, if possible, until pregnancy can be confirmed or ruled out. If the patient does not think she is pregnant, many believe it is advisable to limit the radiation exposure to the first 10 days of the menstrual cycle, if possible, that is, before ovulation and potential conception, particularly if radiologic examination of the abdomen or pelvis is planned. Studies that *must* be done in pregnant women should be performed with careful attention to techniques that reduce the potential risk to the fetus; radiolabeled material that crosses the placental barrier should be particularly avoided.

If doses of irradiation delivered accidentally during pregnancy approach the level of 0.1–0.15 Gy (10–15 rad) to the fetus, an increased incidence of fetal malformations, fetal death, or persistent damage of genetic material in the child may occur, depending on the stage of pregnancy during which the radiation is delivered. The fetus is particularly susceptible to congenital defects during the first trimester of pregnancy.

Consultation with the diagnostic specialist using these tools may help distinguish between the indicated and unwarranted study, as well as assisting in the design, timing, and format of the study to best advantage.

RADIOPHARMACEUTICALS

Compounds linked to a γ-emitting radionuclide may be tailored for concentration by a particular organ or physiologic process. Currently, the radionuclide technetium-99m (^{99m}Tc, where 99 is the atomic weight and m stands for metastable) serves as a label for many radiopharmaceuticals. Technetium-99m is obtained as pertechnetate (TcO_4^-) dissolved in saline solution and is then manipulated to label a wide variety of compounds. A radiopharmaceutical is designated by two parts: the compound and the radionuclide label. Technetium-99m as pertechnetate is useful for imaging thyroid trapping, ^{99m}Tc sulfur colloid for imaging the reticuloendothelial system, and ^{99m}Tc diethylenetriamine-pentaacetic acid (DTPA) for renal imaging.

The chemical quantities of the radionuclide and the pharmaceutical used are generally quite small. Consequently (1) the radiopharmaceuticals do not disturb the process measured, (2) they function as true tracers, and (3) they do not provoke hypersensitivity reactions as do contrast media used in x-ray studies. For example, the amount of iodide used in a thyroid uptake study is thousands of times smaller than that used in ordinary table salt at a meal. The tailoring of the radiopharmaceuticals takes advantage of different processes or properties unique to different organs, as shown in Table 1-1.

Positron-emitting radionuclides of carbon (^{11}C), oxygen (^{15}O), and nitrogen (^{13}N) can be incorporated into a variety of physiologic tracers and substrates, including gaseous oxygen, carbon dioxide, and carbon monoxide. The labeled gases can be used as tracers of the gas itself and, when combined with hemoglobin, as indicators of blood flow, blood volume, and oxygen utilization. Carbohydrates, amino acids, and fatty acids can be synthesized using ^{11}C. In addition, ^{13}N-labeled ammonia can serve as a blood-flow indicator. The half-lives of these radionuclides are in the range of a few minutes, necessitating on-site cyclotron production facilities. As technology advances, the availability of small cyclotrons may become practical for clinical departments. Fluorine-18 (^{18}F) is one positron emitter (half-life of 110 min) that can be made in an off-site production facility and used to label deoxyglucose and other useful substrates. Generator systems that produce rubidium-82 (^{82}Rb) for myocardial imaging studies and gallium-68 (^{68}Ga) for labeling purposes make positron imaging possible without an on-site cyclotron.

An intriguing scanning process, x-ray fluorescence imaging,

uses an external, focused radiation beam of an energy level capable of exciting particular atoms, for example, thyroidal iodine, in order to stimulate them to emit characteristic radiation. Detection of this characteristic radiation offers a method for imaging stable iodine in the thyroid gland. For further discussion, see Chapter 14.

The ability of radiopharmaceuticals to function as indicators of specific physiologic processes provides an important measure of disease that might not be apparent on the basis of structural changes alone. It is the ability of radionuclides to measure function quantitatively and to relate it to structure that is unique to radionuclides in the diagnostic imaging process. Such functional measurements provide a powerful diagnostic tool.

Table 1-1: Radiopharmaceutical Labeling Customized to Cellular Processes

Imaging Objective	Radiopharmaceutical: Mechanism of Localization
Lung scanning	^{99m}Tc albumin macroaggregates or microspheres: capillary blockade
Bone scanning	^{99m}Tc phosphonates: chemiadsorption onto bone crystal
Gastric mucosa uptake as in Meckel's diverticulum imaging, thyroid imaging, salivary imaging	^{99m}Tc pertechnetate: active ion transport
Liver, spleen, and bone marrow imaging	^{99m}Tc sulfur colloid: reticuloendothelial uptake
Hepatocyte and biliary tract imaging	Substituted carbamoyliminodiacetic acid agents: active cellular transport and excretion
Myocardial perfusion and muscle imaging	^{201}Tl, ^{99m}Tc isonitriles, or labeled fatty acids: adenosine triphosphate (ATP) energy-dependent transport system

Table 1-1 *(continued)*

Imaging Objective	Radiopharmaceutical: Mechanism of Localization
Tumor imaging	^{67}Ga citrate: Mechanism of localization in tumors is uncertain Proposed mechanisms: Iron receptor-site binding to facilitate penetration into tumor cells, association with lysozomes intracellularly, reflecting metabolic cell activity ^{111}In, ^{131}I, ^{99m}Tc monoclonal antibodies: immunologic mechanisms
Imaging of infectious/ inflammatory processes	^{67}Ga citrate: Mechanism of localization is uncertain Proposed mechanisms: white blood cell sequestration and/or association with bacterial debris, lactoferrin binding ^{111}In leukocytes: migration of leukocytes to infection/inflammation sites
Brain imaging	^{123}I iodoamphetamine: normal cell perfusion and active organ-specific metabolism; ^{99m}Tc glucoheptonate, ^{99m}Tc DTPA: exclusion by blood-brain barrier except when altered by disease (e.g., tumor, abscess, hematoma, infarct);
Renal imaging and function evaluation	^{99m}Tc DTPA: glomerular filtration and excretion; ^{99m}Tc DMSA: cortical cell uptake; ^{131}I hippuran: renal tubular cell uptake and secretion

IMAGING OF RADIATION

The Anger Scintillation Camera

The most common nuclear medicine studies image the distribution of a radiopharmaceutical in the body with a scintillation or gamma camera. A scintillation camera may be stationary or mobile, that is, capable of being brought to the patient's bedside. It can be designed as a scanning camera that can image the entire body by moving from head to toe. It also can be designed to rotate 360° around the body and, combined with an interfaced dedicated computer, reconstruct tomographic images in any plane (transaxial, coronal, sagittal) using emitted γ-rays (single-photon emission computed tomography) or positrons (positron emission computed tomography). The scintillation camera consists of a detector head and a display console. The detector head of the Anger camera, named for its inventor, Hal Anger, contains a thallium-activated sodium iodide [NaI(Tl)] crystal in a single thin slab of a fixed diameter that can be 25 to 52.5 cm (10 to 21 in.) and a fixed thickness that can be 0.63 to 1.9 cm (¼ to ¾ in.). Other scintillation imaging devices use multiple small crystals.

In the gamma camera, the scintillation crystal absorbs the γ-rays and emits the absorbed energy as a flash or shortly spaced series of flashes of light—scintillations—proportional in brightness to the energy absorbed. Coupled to the crystal is an array of photomultiplier tubes that converts the light flashes originating from the crystal to electronic pulses. An electronic computing circuit sums the outputs of the photomultiplier tubes and assigns an x–y spatial coordinate to the detected γ-ray according to the contribution to the total signal from each PMT in the array. This is translated into voltages applied to the horizontal and vertical plates of a cathode-ray tube (CRT). These voltages position the CRT beam: When it is turned on by detection of an appropriate energy-level pulse, it produces a light flash at a location on the CRT corresponding to the location of interaction of the γ-ray in the crystal. The entire process, from the detection of the γ-ray to the appearance of the light flash on the CRT, requires only $\sim 10^{-5}$ sec. An open-shuttered camera records the separate CRT flashes as dots on film and produces an image of many flashes integrated over a period of time ranging from a fraction of a second to several minutes. Within the limits of motion artifacts and other factors contributing to image degradation, the more counts, or dots, accumulated, the brighter and more detailed the image produced. The degree of film darkening on the image reflects body activity as modified by CRT intensity and camera settings.

γ-Rays emitted from the imaged organ travel radially outward in all directions. A lead or tungsten collimator consisting of a single slab of metal shields the entire crystal. Either many small holes arranged in a parallel, slanted, converging, or diverging array or a single pinhole in the collimator permit the passage of only those γ-rays that are traveling in a direction parallel to the collimator holes, or, in the case of the pinhole collimator, within the angle subtended by the pinhole, through to the crystal. Thus, γ-ray scintillation imaging is an inefficient process. Only a very small fraction of the emitted γ-rays can be used to produce an image.

The data from the camera head may be in either digital or analog form. Analog data may be readily converted to digital form and then stored in a suitable matrix in a computer. Reconstruction of the image from data stored in the computer permits quantitative spatial analysis of the data used to form the image. For example, count rate changes in a particular region may be determined and related to a physiologic process.

POSITRON EMISSION TOMOGRAPHY

Positron emission tomography (PET), one of the fastest-growing areas in nuclear medicine, is a technique for making tomographic images of the distribution of positron-emitting radioactive tracers in the body. Such images show physiologic and biochemical processes, while computed tomography (CT) and magnetic resonance (MRI) images show mainly morphology or chemical constituency. Through PET, in vivo physiology and biochemistry are imaged. The observation that many morphologic images of x-ray, CT, ultrasound, and MRI could be obtained in a cadaver, while PET studies like all nuclear medicine studies require a living organism dramatizes the essential difference between the functional images of PET studies and other imaging methods.

Positrons (positive electrons) are emitted from proton excess radioactive nuclei, and travel only a few millimeters in tissue before colliding with a negative electron. This encounter results in the annihilation of both particles, with the creation of two γ-rays of 511 keV each, the energy equivalent of the two electron masses. These annihilation photons travel in 180° opposite directions.

Positron detectors detect the pair of γ-rays resulting from the positron–electron annihilation. The detectors are placed on opposite sides of the positron source to be imaged and only register a count if both detect a photon at precisely the same time, a coincidence event. A modern PET camera is a system of many detectors, dozens to several hundred, placed in a circular or polygonal arrangement surrounding the patient who has received a positron-emitting radionuclide. Electronic circuits and computers pair off detectors to register in a coincidence mode. A detector on one side of the body is paired to count in coincidence with detectors on the opposite side of the body. Two paired detectors on opposite sides of the body that detect a photon simultaneously—a coincidence event—establish a line along which the source must lie. Filters and other computer-controlled image manipulation techniques are then used to reconstruct a cross-sectional image from this information.

PET cameras may have many rings of detectors; coincidence circuits can pair up not only the detectors in any one ring, but detectors in adjacent rings as well. Thus, an eight-ring system can generate images of 15 slices simultaneously with each image containing several million counts. Images can be obtained at rates of up to several per second, permitting the study of dynamic processes. The data-processing requirements for such a system are staggering. Collimation problems inherent in single photon imaging are not a concern in positron imaging. Attenuation changes can be corrected for by appropriate calculations using calibration studies. These characteristics of PET imaging permit generation of quantitative data concerning radioisotope distribution.

As noted in the section on radiopharmaceuticals, the positron-emitting radionuclides are elements of great biologic interest. With the exception of ^{18}F, because of its 2-hr half-life, and a few generator systems (e.g., ^{82}Rb and ^{68}Ga), use of other positron-emitting radionuclides requires an on-site cyclotron. Because of the rapid decay of most positron emitters, preparing the tracers in their desired form (e.g., glucose or dopamine) for biomedical use demands rapid synthetic techniques. In 1986 more than 300 substances and drugs labeled with positron emitting radionuclides had been described and the list is growing. The final form of positron-labeled radiopharmaceuticals is often piped from the cyclotron area where rapid or automated chemical synthesis is performed, directly to the patient who is in position in the PET camera. Because of the short tracer half-life, repeat studies can be done a few minutes later, permitting evaluation of drug or other intervention.

Chapter 5 on the heart and Chapter 12 on the central nervous system present some examples of PET imaging illustrating its unique ability to provide insights into organ function and metabolism. With unlimited potential for the development of new tracers, PET has a promising future, particularly when coupled with lower costs and easier operation of the medical cyclotrons. It is important to recognize that PET is much more than an imaging modality, and that its power lies in its ability to give absolute quantification of local blood flow and metabolic activity, and unique information about physiologic and biochemical body functions.

SINGLE-PHOTON EMISSION COMPUTED TOMOGRAPHY

Single-photon emission computed tomography (SPECT) uses the gamma scintillation camera that is currently widely available for clinical use. In SPECT, like CT, data (emitted photons in SPECT, transmitted x-rays in CT) are taken from multiple angles, usually encompassing 180° or 360°, around the body and used for computer reconstruction of multiple tomograms. Tomographic images are reconstructed in coronal, sagittal, and transverse projections. This approach provides increased contrast as well as better anatomical delineation than is possible with planar imaging. The ability to quantitate tracer distribution is not as good as with PET because of problems of collimation and attenuation, which are inherent in the detection of single photons. Nonetheless, with the development of new compounds which can be labeled with currently available single-photon emitters such as ^{99m}Tc and ^{123}I, SPECT provides a means for qualitatively investigating metabolic and physiologic processes such as myocardial blood flow and cerebral perfusion and applying them clinically. Examples of these uses in clinical practice are illustrated in Chapter 5 (heart) and Chapter 12 (brain).

SELECTED READINGS

Radiation

Brill AB (ed). *Low-level radiation effects: A fact book.* New York: Society of Nuclear Medicine; 1983

Cohn HI, Fry RJM. Radiation carcinogenesis. *N Engl J Med* 1984; 310:504–511

NCRP. *Basic radiation protection criteria.* NCRP Rept No 39. Washington, DC: National Council on Radiation Protection and Measurements; 1980

NCRP. *Natural background radiation in the United States.* NCRP Rept No 45. Washington, DC: National Council on Radiation Protection and Measurements; 1975

Noz ME, Maguire GQ Jr. *Radiation protection in the radiologic and health sciences.* 2nd ed. Philadelphia: Lea & Febiger; 1985

Radiopharmaceuticals

Heindel ND, Gurns HD, Schneider R, Foster NI. Principles of rational radiopharmaceutical design. In: Spencer RP, ed. *Radiophar-*

maceuticals: Structure-activity relationships. New York: Grune & Stratton; 1981:101–127

Phan T, Wasnich R. *Practical nuclear pharmacy.* 2nd ed. Honolulu: Banyan Enterprises, Ltd; 1981

Subramanian G, Rhodes BA, Cooper JF, Sodd VJ (eds). *Radiopharmaceuticals.* New York: Society of Nuclear Medicine; 1975

Instrumentation

Parker RP, Smith PHS, Taylor DM. *Basic science of nuclear medicine.* 2nd ed. New York: Churchill Livingston; 1984:167–271

Reivich M, Alavi A (eds). *Positron emission tomography.* New York: Alan R. Liss; 1985

Sorenson JA, Phelps ME. *Physics in nuclear medicine.* 2nd ed. New York: Grune & Stratton; 1987:298–361, 424–451

2

The Diagnostic Process and Nuclear Medicine

Test results provide a measurement to aid the physician in estimating diagnostic probabilities. The physician must understand what the test actually measures in order to interpret the results. Three things must be known for proper interpretation of a test result: test sensitivity, test specificity, and the prior probability, that is, the probability of the presence of disease before doing the test. Test sensitivity and specificity for a particular disease or process are available from the medical literature.

Physicians should be aware, however, that often the reported sensitivity and specificity are obtained from evaluations of a new test carried out by investigators with a keen interest and expertise in the disease being investigated by the new test. Using their expertise, they carefully select the group to which they apply the new measurement and a control group. The prevalence of disease in these study groups and how the presence or absence of disease in these groups is ultimately determined, and particularly whether the results of the test being evaluated enter into the decision to further study these groups, prove critical in determining test sensitivity and specificity. In the following discussion, it is assumed for simplicity that a test result is either positive or negative and that the result is either true or false. Because the limits of normal may be altered to affect test sensitivity and specificity and there is an overlap between values in a control population and those with disease, these assumptions are not correct in practice.

SENSITIVITY, SPECIFICITY, AND RECEIVER OPERATING CHARACTERISTIC CURVE

Sensitivity measures the ability of a test to detect a disease when it is present. It is the ratio of true positive (TP) results compared with all those with disease—true-positive (TP) and false-negative (FN) results. This may be abbreviated as:

$$\text{Sensitivity} = \frac{TP}{TP + FN}$$

Sensitivity of a test may be increased by changing the cutoff value between what is considered normal and what is considered abnormal. Since there is a spread of results in a "normal" population, usually described by a bell-shaped curve, normal values at either end of the spectrum usually overlap the population of abnormal individuals.

   The physician who interprets an image visually may consciously or subconsciously alter this cutoff point. For example, in interpretation of a bone scan of a child suspected of having osteomyelitis, the observer will often skew the interpretation to increase sensitivity by applying liberal criteria of slight asymmetry for interpreting the image as abnormal. The result is an increase in the false-positive results, which is justifiable if one considers the morbidity that may result if the diagnosis is not made and appropriate treatment is not instituted in a timely fashion. If the clinician considers the bone scan as a screening procedure and would not appropriately pursue the diagnosis in a child with a normal bone scan, then weighing this error against overtreating a child who may have only a soft tissue infection, but not osteomyelitis, will lead to such an approach. Furthermore, the positive outcome will often be followed by further diagnostic investigations such as magnetic resonance imaging or a more invasive procedure such as needle aspiration to confirm the diagnosis. Some normal individuals will be subjected to these procedures with a concomitant increase in risk and increased expense with the justification that no one who really needs treatment will be missed.

Specificity measures the ability to exclude disease when it is absent. It is the ratio of true negative (TN) results to all those without disease—true-negative (TN) and false-positive (FP) results. It may be expressed as

$$\text{Specificity} = \frac{TN}{TN + FP}$$

In the example above, increasing the sensitivity of the bone scan by applying liberal criteria for abnormality leads to decreased specificity, or an increase in the false-positive results. Specificity can be increased by the interpreter employing strict criteria for what is considered abnormal and increasing the limits of what is accepted as normal. For example, in interpreting the liver scan, the interpreter may purposely choose to increase the specificity based on the following two considerations. If the liver scan is read as abnormal, the clinician who has been searching for metastatic disease often accepts the abnormal liver scan as sufficient evidence that metastatic disease is present. This could be a grave error that could cost the patient a chance for appropriate treatment and cure. A false-negative liver scan interpretation may have a less drastic effect although it may cause the patient to undergo unnecessary treatment. The metastatic disease will become evident if present in spite of the liver scan interpretation.

The relationship between the true-positive fraction (sensitivity) and the false-positive fraction (1−specificity) established by plotting one against the other for varying criteria for abnormality, forms a receiver operating characteristic (ROC) curve shown in Fig. 2-1. The ROC curve shows that for a given test and varying interpretative criteria, strict or liberal, the observer can increase sensitivity only at the expense of specificity. In attempting to increase sensitivity to include all those with disease, the observer invariably classifies a greater fraction of those without disease as having disease. Attempts to segregate out all

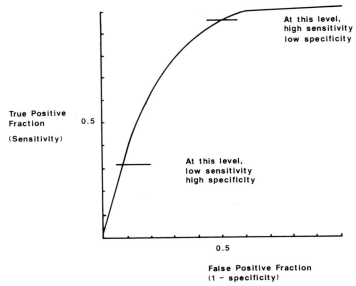

FIG. 2-1. Receiver operating characteristic curve is a plot of observer sensitivity, the true-positive fraction of results against the false-positive fraction of results or nonspecificity (1 − specificity) on using different criteria, strict as opposed to liberal for interpreting a study. It shows that in using strict criteria there is low sensitivity but high specificity. When liberal criteria are used, the sensitivity increases but specificity falls.

normals by increasing interpretative specificity will lead to decreased sensitivity.

PREDICTIVE VALUE, PREVALENCE, AND BAYES' THEOREM

Prior probability, that is, the probability that the patient had the disease (D+) prior to performing the test has a great influence in determining what the odds are of a patient with a positive test result having disease (the positive predictive value of the test). Without an estimate of the prior probability, the probability that a patient has a disease cannot be determined from the test result. This is one of the most poorly understood concepts of the diagnostic process.

The clinician should ask the question, "Given a positive test, what is the probability of the patient having the disease?" or, "Given a negative test, what is the likelihood that the patient does not have the disease?" Bayes formulated a theorem that permits one to answer these questions by estimating the predictive value of a test. The positive predictive value is the ratio of true-positive results to all positive results. The negative predictive value is the ratio of true-negative results to all negative results. In order to estimate the predictive value, the final step in the diagnostic process, one needs to know the prevalence of disease (D+) in the population to which the test is applied. If the total population is 1, the fraction without disease is (1 − D+).

The numerator for a test result's positive predictive value—true-positive results—equals the test sensitivity times disease prevalence in the population to which the patient belongs before running the test. The denominator, all positive test results, is the true-positive results added to the false-positive results. The false-positive results are obtained by multiplying the nonspecificity of the test (1 − specificity) times the nondisease prevalence (1 − prevalence). This can be summed up as follows:

$$\text{Positive predictive value} = \frac{TP}{TP + FP}$$

$$= \frac{\text{Sensitivity} \times (D+)}{\text{Sensitivity} \times (D+) + (1 - \text{specificity}) \times (1 - D+)}$$

$$\text{Negative predictive value} = \frac{TN}{TN + FN}$$

$$= \frac{\text{Specificity} \times (1 - D+)}{\text{Specificity} \times (1 - D+) + (1 - \text{sensitivity}) \times (D+)}$$

For the positive predictive value, the numerator depends not only on test sensitivity, but also on the estimated disease prevalence, D+. If the prevalence is very low, then the value of the numerator falls, as does the positive predictive value.

To illustrate this point, we will use a clinical example, the two-stage Schilling test for measuring the absorption of vitamin B_{12}, a test that is 100% sensitive and 95% specific for diagnosing pernicious anemia. Yet despite its high sensitivity and specificity, the value of this test in practice is highly dependent on the population to which we apply the test. The test is not very helpful if we apply it to a population in which the prevalence of pernicious anemia is quite low. Although there is some debate about the true prevalence of pernicious anemia in blacks, with evidence of increasing incidence in young black women, for the purpose of this example, we will assume a prevalence of pernicious anemia of 1 in 10,000 in blacks with anemia. For every 100 people in this population who do not have pernicious anemia, we will find 5 positive tests since 95% specificity means there will be a 5% false-positive result. By the time we screen 10,000 such patients to find the one that does have pernicious anemia, we will have found ~500 false-positive test results for every true-positive result. Thus, for any given positive result in this population, the odds that the individual actually has the disease are ~1 in 500. Admittedly the odds of 1 in 500 are better than 1 in 10,000, but application of the test to this population has not improved the odds enough to arrive at a diagnosis. Why not? The reason lies not in a faulty test, but in faulty application of a very good test to a population with a low prior probability of having the disease being sought. These results point out that the indiscriminant application of even a very "good" test to an inappropriate population is not helpful. The physician must screen the population before using the test to aid in diagnosis. The screening must be done by appropriate intelligent use of the history and physical examination data as well as independent laboratory results.

The effect of disease prevalence on the positive predictive value of a test can also be seen from the following example using planar thallium stress myocardial imaging with a sensitivity of 80% and a specificity of 90% for coronary artery disease. In a low-prevalence population (e.g., nonsmoking, nonhypertensive women in their fourth decade with atypical chest pain), let us estimate the prevalence of significant coronary artery disease at 10%. Of 1000 such individuals, 100 would be expected to have significant coronary artery disease and the following analysis applies:

	Disease Present D+	Disease Absent D−
	100	900
Thallium stress test positive T^+	80	90
Thallium stress test negative T^-	20	810
	80% sensitive	90% specific

$$\text{Positive predictive value} = \frac{\text{true-positive results}}{\text{all positive results}} = \frac{80}{170} = 47\%$$

$$\text{Negative predictive value} = \frac{\text{true-negative results}}{\text{all negative results}} = \frac{810}{830} = 98\%$$

These calculations show that in this low-prevalence population, a patient with a positive thallium stress test would have only a 1 in 2 probability of having significant coronary artery disease. But, if the test were negative, the probability of having significant coronary artery disease would be almost nil. In this population, a negative test would have most value. If we apply exactly the same test to another population of patients with a 50% prevalence of coronary artery disease, for example a sedentary group of hypertensive men in their fourth decade who smoke and experience chest pain after heavy meals, the predictive values are entirely different:

	Disease Present D+	Disease Absent D−
	500	500
Thallium stress test positive T^+	400	50
Thallium stress test negative T^-	100	450
	80% sensitive	90% specific

$$\text{Positive predictive value} = \frac{\text{true-positive results}}{\text{all positive results}} = \frac{400}{450} = 89\%$$

$$\text{Negative predictive value} = \frac{\text{true-negative results}}{\text{all negative results}} = \frac{450}{550} = 82\%$$

These calculations show that a positive thallium stress test result in this population would raise the probability of having significant coronary artery disease to nine in ten. Similarly a negative thallium stress test indicates a four in five chance of not having significant coronary artery disease.

These results emphasize that a test result can have a much different value, depending on independently assessed probabilities before the test is performed. In the first low-prevalence population, a negative thallium stress test appears valuable, virtually excluding disease. The positive test result in this population is less valuable. In the second moderate prevalence group, the probability is altered from even odds to a nine in ten chance of having the disease if the test is positive and a four in five chance of not having the disease if the test is negative.

Is this alteration of probabilities sufficient to justify performing the test? The answer depends on many factors including economic considerations, patient attitude, presence of skill and facilities to perform coronary angiography, and the availability of therapy and desire to use it on the part of those involved in the decision-making process. What is critical to the diagnostic process is that the physician understand the effect of prior probability on the diagnostic value of a test result.

A graphic solution to Bayes' theorem is shown in Fig. 2-2. The graph relates post-test probability to pretest probability for a positive result (positive predictive value) of a sensitive and fairly specific test. The plot shows that if the pretest probability is low, at point A, the post-test probability cannot be sufficient to establish the diagnosis. As the pretest probability increases to point B, so does the positive predictive value of a positive test outcome.

The message is: Don't use a laboratory test without having some estimate of the presence of disease in the patient before

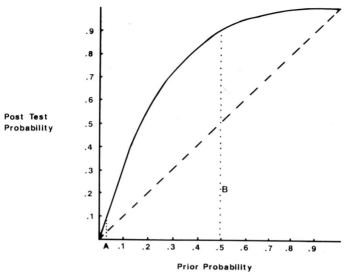

Post Test Probability

Prior Probability

FIG. 2-2. Graphic solution to Bayes' theorem for a sensitive and relatively specific test. It relates pretest probability of having the disease to post-test probability of having the disease. At point A, the probability of having the disease prior to the test is 2% (0.02), and a positive test result has a 10% (0.1) positive predictive value or probability of actually being due to disease. At point B, with a 50% (0.5) prior probability, a positive test result has a 90% (0.9) positive predictive value. The dashed line shows the plot of a worthless test that does not alter the prior probabilities.

doing the test. Otherwise, the significance of the test result will be uncertain. Before you perform a test, have in mind what course of action you will follow if the test is positive and what course you will take if it is negative. If the test will make no difference in choosing a course of treatment, the test is probably superfluous.

Tests are most helpful when they alter prior probabilities the most. In general, this occurs when prior probabilities are ~50/50. Sensitive tests are usually most useful when the outcome is normal, thereby virtually excluding disease. For example, a normal perfusion lung scan makes pulmonary embolic disease extremely unlikely. By contrast, when positive, a sensitive test may yield little information on the exact cause of the abnormality and additional relevant data from other independent tests will be required. Specific tests are most helpful when they are abnormal, thereby virtually ensuring the presence of disease.

Nuclear medicine procedures are generally sensitive measures of some physiologic function, often portrayed with anatomic features. They are frequently most useful when normal. The images provide a means of mapping and tracing physiologic processes. The physical process of detecting radioactive decay is inherently quantitative, since discrete events are counted in the detection process. Tracers, by definition, do not alter the process they are used to measure, so that data derived from such procedures are free from distortion caused by the test itself.

Furthermore, disturbance in process rates may be the initial manifestation of disease. Such changes may be detectable by quantitative methods prior to the gross changes of decompensated disease. There are abundant examples of the body's ability to compensate for abnormal states. For example, protein loss through the gut can be compensated for by increasing the rate of hepatic protein synthesis. This adjustment may result in a normal serum albumin level, but measurement of protein loss in the stool, or protein turnover rates or imaging the abdomen after intravenous injection of radiolabeled albumin will indicate the true state of affairs.

Radionuclide methodology offers a unique means of investigating ongoing physiologic processes. The fact that in many cases the study provides an anatomic image should not obscure the fact that a physiologic process is being measured. When obtaining a nuclear medicine study, it is helpful to understand what the test actually measures and how this measurement can be integrated into the diagnostic process.

SELECTED READINGS

Diamond GA, Forrester JS. Analysis of probability as an aid in the clinical diagnosis of coronary-artery disease. *N Engl J Med* 1979; 300:1350–1358

Goris ML. *Sensitivities and specificities of scintigraphic procedures.* Chicago: Year Book Medical Publishers; 1985

Griner PF, Mayewski RJ, Mushlin AI, et al. Selection and interpretation of diagnostic tests and procedures: Principles and applications. *Ann Intern Med* 1981; 94(part 2):553–600

Hamilton GW, Trobaugh GB, Ritchie JL, et al. Myocardial imaging with Tl-201: An analysis of clinical usefulness based on Bayes' theorem. *Semin Nucl Med* 1978; 8:358–364

McNeil BJ, Keeler E, Adelstein SJ. Primer on certain elements of medical decision making. *N Engl J Med* 1975; 293:211–215

Patton DD. Introduction to clinical decision making. *Semin Nucl Med* 1978; 8:273–282

Pauker SG, Kassier JP. Therapeutic decision making: A cost benefit analysis. *N Engl J Med* 1975; 293:229–234

Rozanski A, Berman D. The efficacy of cardiovascular nuclear medicine exercise studies. *Semin Nucl Med* 1987; 17:104–120

Organ Imaging with Radionuclides

3
Endocrinology

THYROID UPTAKE AND IMAGING

Thyroid hormone biosynthesis begins when inorganic plasma iodide is trapped by the thyroid gland. Oxidation of iodide to iodine and organification follow. The iodine substitutes onto the tyrosyl rings linked to thyroglobulin, a glycoprotein stored within the follicular lumen. These iodotyrosines then couple, forming iodothyronines—the thyroid hormones, triiodothyronine (T_3) and thyroxine or tetraiodothyronine (T_4). The iodothyronines are split from thyroglobulin and are secreted as the thyroid hormones. T_3 and T_4 circulate in blood, chiefly bound to serum proteins. Free T_3 and free T_4, the only active forms of thyroid hormone, represent ~0.5% of the total circulating thyroid hormones.

Radioactive Iodine Uptake

The radioactive iodine uptake study is performed by oral administration of a radioisotope of iodine, usually iodine-123 (^{123}I) or ^{131}I, to the fasting patient (since food slows absorption), followed by measurement of the uptake in the neck at an early interval varying from 2–6 hr and again at 24 hr. The counts in the thyroid are compared with a standard of the administered dose; the percentage taken up by the thyroid is then calculated.

The thyroidal radioactive iodine uptake (RAIU) provides an index of thyroid trapping and organification of iodide measured as a percentage of administered iodide taken up by the gland. It depends not only on thyroid function, but on the body's iodide pool as well. In effect, for a larger iodide pool, a smaller percentage of the administered radioactive iodide will be trapped by the gland in fulfilling the thyroidal iodide requirement for hormonal biosynthesis.

Many sources of iodide expand the iodide pool, particularly the organic iodides used for radiographic contrast in excretory urography, computed tomographic (CT) scanning, angiography, cholecystography, cholangiography, myelography, and lymphangiography. The latter two procedures leave organic sources of iodide that can expand the inorganic iodide pool for months to years. Dietary sources of iodide pool expansion, chiefly the periodate used as a preservative by bakers, also reduce the percentage of thyroidal uptake of radioiodine.

Because of these nearly ubiquitous sources of iodide and the fact that it is only an indirect measure of thyroid function, the RAIU should not be used to evaluate whether a patient is euthyroid. Measuring circulating levels of thyroid hormone (as discussed in Nonimaging Procedures, Chapter 14) not only provides the most accurate assessment of overall thyroid function, but involves no patient irradiation. The RAIU is best reserved to answer certain specific questions concerning thyroid function: Is there an organification defect in thyroid hormone production? Is the gland taking up an adequate percentage of administered iodide to make therapy with radioiodine feasible? Is hyperthyroidism caused by a disorder associated with a low uptake, such as subacute thyroiditis, struma ovarii, or factitious hyperthyroidism?

TSH Stimulation and Suppression

The response of thyroidal uptake to thyroid-stimulating hormone (TSH) or thyrotropin-releasing hormone (TRH) can be helpful in evaluating the thyroid–pituitary–hypothalamic servomechanism. The TSH or TRH stimulation test can be used together with thyroid imaging to (1) identify normal-functioning thyroid tissue suppressed by hyperfunctioning tissue, (2) help identify functioning metastases from differentiated thyroid carcinoma, and (3) assess thyroid functional reserve after a baseline study. Normally, the RAIU is increased at least 33% by TSH.

Thyroid suppression studies evaluate the response of the thyroid gland or a functioning thyroid nodule to the removal of the endogenous TSH signal. The classic findings of Graves' disease—hyperthyroidism, goiter, ophthalmopathy, and dermopathy—may not always be present in a patient. Even though in some cases the gland may not produce enough thyroid hormone to render the patient clearly hyperthyroid, the gland will always operate autonomously in this disease, that is, its ability to produce thyroid hormone is independent of TSH. The TSH suppression study evaluates whether the thyroid gland functions independently of circulating TSH levels. The suppression study is performed by administering sufficient exogenous thyroid hormone, either triiodothyronine (T_3) or thyroxine (T_4), to suppress pituitary TSH secretion over a 10-day period and then repeating either the image or the uptake or both and comparing it with the baseline study. Uptake normally decreases by 50% or more.

Perchlorate Washout Test

The perchlorate washout test evaluates whether thyroidal organification of iodide is proceeding normally. This function may be impaired in congenital goiters and is commonly impaired in Hashimoto's thyroiditis. Iodide taken up by the thyroid becomes bound within minutes to the thyroglobulin molecule. If the trapping mechanism gradient is overwhelmed with perchlorate, the trapped iodide already bound to thyroglobulin will remain in the gland, whereas any iodide that has not been organified will leak out. A significant fall in the activity in the thyroid gland after administration of a large dose of perchlorate indicates failure of organification of trapped iodide.

Thyroid Imaging

Thyroid imaging with radionuclides provides a means of visualizing functional morphology. Radioisotopes of iodide may be used,

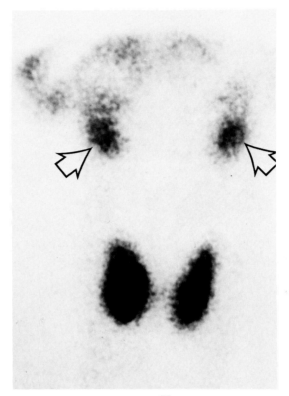

FIG. 3-1. Normal thyroid image with ^{99m}Tc pertechnetate shows uniform trapping of activity in proportion to gland volume. Activity can be seen in the salivary glands, above (*arrows* indicate submandibular glands). Slight soft tissue activity may also be seen.

as may the anion analogue of iodide, pertechnetate, which is trapped but not organified (Fig. 3-1). Technetium-99m pertechnetate and ^{123}I are the preferred radionuclides for thyroid imaging. Iodine-131, although used occasionally in small doses of 5–10 µCi for thyroid uptake determinations, is not recommended as an imaging agent, except for ectopic thyroid searches, because its emission of a 360-keV photon is imaged very inefficiently and with poor resolution by the scintillation camera. In addition, for imaging, large doses [3.7 MBq (100 µCi)] are needed, which give unacceptably high radiation doses to the thyroid gland if thyroid uptake is high or normal. Technetium-99m or ^{123}I gives 1–10% of the radiation dose of ^{131}I, or usually only 0.01–0.02 Gy (1–2 rad) to the thyroid gland. Both have favorable photon emissions for high-resolution images with the scintillation camera.

Thyroid Nodules

Occasional reports of discordant images between ^{123}I and ^{99m}Tc pertechnetate relative to thyroid nodules have appeared in the literature. This finding may be explained by the fact that pertechnetate reflects only trapping and is imaged within 30 min of intravenous administration, whereas the iodide distribution reflects both trapping and organification and is usually imaged 6–24 hr after oral administration. Areas that trap but that do not organify the ion may appear to have good function with pertechnetate, but poor function with iodide. The division of thyroid nodules into hyperfunctioning (hot) (see Fig. 3-2), normally functioning, and nonfunctioning (cold) (see Fig. 3-3) by imaging has been made on the basis of experience accumulated with images performed 24 hr after administration of radioactive ^{131}I. The classification is important, since reports of skillfully screened populations indicate that 15–20% of cold nodules may be malignant and therefore warrant biopsy, whereas hot nodules almost always are benign.

Thyroid imaging provides a means of documenting the location, size, shape, and functional characteristics of thyroid tissue. For unknown reasons, goiters, that is, enlarged thyroid glands, may be associated with multiple thyroid lumps called nodules. Iodide deficiency, a rare finding in the United States, may cause nontoxic goiters; that is, the patient is not hyperthyroid. Frequent ingestion of certain foods such as rutabagas and turnips may have the same effect. Growth stimulating antibodies have been found in some patients. Images show an enlarged gland with uneven function and lack of responsiveness to TSH.

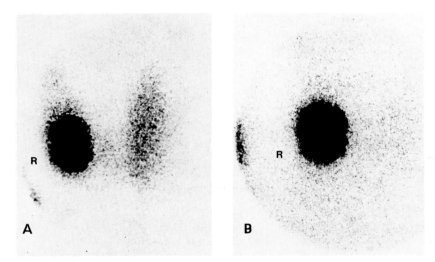

FIG. 3-2. Hyperfunctioning ("hot") nodule in the middle of the right lobe of the thyroid (**A**), which is not producing sufficient thyroid hormone to shut off thyroid-stimulating hormone (TSH). This is evident from the visualization of the normal left lobe and upper part of the right lobe. After suppression with thyroid hormone, a repeat image (**B**) shows that the entire gland is shut off except for the autonomous nodule. Such lumps are almost always benign. The radioisotope used is ^{99m}Tc pertechnetate.

Ectopic Thyroid Tissue

In two-thirds of cases, congenital, sporadic hypothyroidism is associated with poorly functioning thyroidal tissue, often in ectopic position. Hereditable hypothyroidism is usually associated with a normally positioned gland, often with increased trapping. Pertechnetate images help identify those infants who might have this disorder. Thyroglossal duct cysts rarely concentrate iodide or pertechnetate. Their diagnosis therefore depends on palpation of a midline neck mass. In some cases, anterior mediastinal masses may be caused by substernal extension of thyroid tissue. Imaging over the mediastinum after radioactive iodine administration confirms the diagnosis of this condition. Rarely, ectopic thyroid tissue may function autonomously, caus-

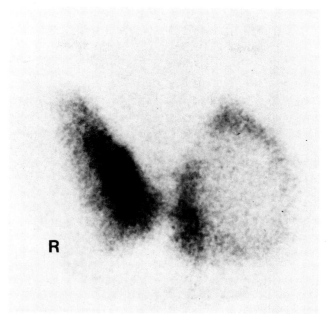

FIG. 3-3. Nonfunctioning ("cold") thyroid nodule expanding the left thyroid lobe. This nonspecific finding is shared by benign and malignant neoplasms and a variety of other causes of thyroidal lumps. The radioisotope used is [123]I.

ing hyperthyroidism. This finding occurs in so-called struma ovarii—ectopic thyroid tissue in the ovaries. Thyroid tissue in ectopic sites is subject to all the diseases of a normally situated thyroid.

Abnormalities of the Thyroid Gland

Toxic goiters causing hyperthyroidism include the hyperplastic, hyperfunctioning gland associated with Graves' disease (diffuse toxic goiter) and uninodular and multinodular toxic goiter, in which hyperfunctioning areas may suppress more normally responsive tissue. These hyperfunctioning nodules are not malignant.

Nonfunctioning (cold) thyroid nodules may represent benign adenomas, cysts, hemorrhage, focal thyroiditis, malignant neoplasm, metastasis, or abscess. Ultrasound can be used to distinguish cystic from solid nodules. Histologic verification is the only means of definitively distinguishing thyroid malignancy from the many other causes of cold nodules.

Acute suppurative thyroiditis is a clinical rarity. Subacute thyroiditis is usually a painful, self-limited, often recrudescent problem believed to be of viral origin. In this disease, disruption of thyroidal follicles interferes with iodide uptake and may also release enough preformed hormone into the bloodstream to cause transient thyrotoxicosis. Generally, the images produced in this disorder show either nonvisualization of the thyroid or uneven function. Hashimoto's thyroiditis is a chronic, painless lymphocytic infiltration of the thyroid tissue that causes an organification defect early in its course. Eventually, the thyroid functional reserve decreases, although the patient may still be euthyroid. Finally, hypothyroidism may supervene. Images early in the disease may show an enlarged gland with normal or increased trapping. Later, function and morphology may appear markedly uneven.

RADIOIODINE THERAPY

Iodine-131 given in doses 100–2000 times diagnostic tracer doses can be used to treat benign and malignant thyroid disease. The β-radiation given off by ^{131}I is effective in irradiating the immediate local region of tissue in which the ^{131}I is concentrated, since β-radiation is able to travel only millimeters in tissue. β-Radiation is used most often to treat the hyperthyroidism associated with Graves' disease in nonpregnant adults. Hypothyroidism is a common sequela of this therapy, but it is also seen frequently in patients treated surgically and in those maintained on long-term antithyroid medication. Hypothyroidism appears to represent an end point of the natural course of the disease. Radioiodine therapy is less expensive and does not carry the immediate, but low incidence of morbidity associated with surgery, such as recurrent laryngeal nerve injury with vocal cord paralysis and hypoparathyroidism from inadvertent injury to or removal of parathyroids.

Less frequently, radioiodide is used to treat toxic nodular goiters, since such glands are often quite large and have less avidity for iodide. These glands require the administration of higher doses of radioiodine to achieve euthyroidism. The radiation exposure to the normal thyroid tissue in these patients is minimal because its function is suppressed by the high levels of endogenous thyroid hormone.

THYROID CARCINOMA

Complete surgical removal of neoplasm is the basic principle for treating differentiated thyroid cancer. Statistics suggest that survival is improved if large ablative doses of 3.7–5.6 GBq (100–150 mCi) of ^{131}I are given to destroy any residual functioning thyroid tissue in differentiated thyroid carcinoma, follicular, papillary, mixed papillary–follicular, and an occasional Hürthle cell carcinoma that concentrates radioiodine. Subsequent doses are given when indicated. Usually, at 4–6 wk post-thyroidectomy, a whole-body thyroid scan is performed to detect metastases and residual functioning thyroid tissue. Therapeutic ^{131}I doses of 3.7–5.6 GBq (100–150 mCi) are administered to eradicate tumor or residual functioning thyroid tissue if the scan shows uptake in such regions. Whole-body ^{131}I scans in search of metastases are generally repeated at 6-mo or annual intervals, followed by repeat therapy doses of ^{131}I when warranted. Optimization of ^{131}I localization in functioning thyroid tissue or tumor is achieved if ^{131}I uptake can be stimulated by a rise in endogenous TSH or exogenous TSH. In addition to whole-body imaging, functioning metastases may be detected by following thyroglobulin levels in the hypothyroid state. Radiation thyroiditis and sialitis may be seen as complications of these megadoses. The most serious reported complication of multiple therapies with cumulative doses of 15–30 GBq (500–1000 mCi) is leukemia from excessive bone marrow radiation. Radiation safety measures must be carefully adhered to when these large doses of ^{131}I are used.

PARATHYROID IMAGING

The plethora of imaging tests that have been developed for detecting hyperfunctioning parathyroid tissue testifies to the lack of the surgeon's confidence in any single method to guide in the search for the source of excess parathormone production. The skilled surgeon will find the source better than 90% of the time on initial exploration but is successful <75% of the time in cases involving re-exploration. Since the distinction between adenomas and hyperplasia may not be evident prior to surgery, and hyperfunctioning adenomas may be small, multiple, and even ectopic (being found in the mediastinum on occasion), an accurate means of localization would shorten the surgical time and increase the success rate of re-exploration.

Thallium–technetium pertechnetate subtraction imaging has proved very helpful for this purpose. Thallium is localized in a variety of benign and malignant neoplasms through as yet imperfectly understood mechanisms. Since thallium acts as a potassium analogue, thallium uptake in neoplasms may be related to transmembrane potential generated by cellular ATP-dependent sodium/potassium pump mechanisms. Such uptake is independent of hormone synthetic mechanisms. Technetium pertechnetate uptake in the neck region is chiefly related to the thyroid trapping mechanism for anions. Thus thallium uptake in an area in which there is no pertechnetate trapping indicates the presence of tissue other than normal thyroid, such as parathyroid adenoma or hyperplasia. Normally functioning parathyroid glands are not detectable by this technique. Unfortunately, however, this property is not unique to hyperfunctioning parathyroid tissue, and thallium–technetium pertechnetate subtraction imaging can be positive in other conditions, including benign or malignant thyroidal or extrathyroidal neoplasms that occur in the neck.

Thallium–technetium pertechnetate subtraction imaging is used for localizing hyperfunctioning parathyroid tissue, once the biochemical diagnosis of primary hyperparathyroidism has been made. The imaging technique can identify either a single adenoma, multiple adenomas, ectopic adenomas, or hyperplastic glands. Thallium–pertechnetate imaging has proved both valuable and practical, since it can be applied to nonhospitalized patients without any special preparation and without any serious risk.

Images of the neck and upper mediastinum as well as computer-stored information are obtained over a 10-min period following the administration of thallium-201 (^{201}Tl), which emits low-energy photons ranging from 69 to 83 keV, with less abundant photons at 135 and 167 keV. Without moving the patient, ^{99m}Tc pertechnetate, which emits a higher-energy photon of 140 keV and is trapped only in the thyroid gland, is administered; again, data from the neck and upper mediastinum are stored in an on-line computer for image analysis. Since the energies of ^{201}Tl and ^{99m}Tc are very different, their distributions are readily separated by collecting data from electronically different windows set to accept only selected energy levels. Computer-controlled subtraction is then performed. This permits detection of regions of excess thallium uptake over pertechnetate trapping. Often, computer subtraction is not necessary to detect excess thallium accumulation, but sometimes it is the only means by which such tissue can be demonstrated. Color-coded subtraction appears helpful in emphasizing small areas of discordant thallium concentration.

Approximately 80% of parathyroid adenomas can be localized by this means. While some investigators have reported a similar success rate with parathyroid hyperplasia, others have not. This may relate to the larger size of the adenoma as compared with the hyperplastic gland at the time of diagnosis. Scintigraphic detectability depends on size, with the limits ranging from 300 to 800 mg, as well as the ability of the tissue to concentrate thallium. The technique may be less accurate in the neck that has already been explored. Figure 3-4 demonstrates localization of a single parathyroid adenoma using this tech-

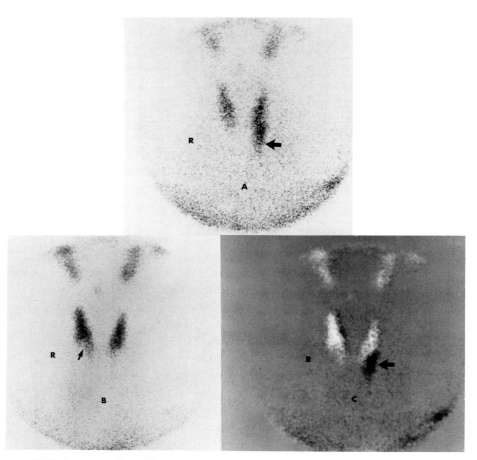

FIG. 3-4. Parathyroid adenoma visualized by thallium–technetium per-technetate subtraction imaging. (**A**) Image with ^{201}Tl shows extension of tissue downward from the inferior aspect of the left thyroid lobe (*solid arrow*). (**B**) The technetium-99m pertechnetate image shows no trapping in this area. In addition, a small intrathyroidal defect can be seen in the right lobe of the thyroid (*small arrow*), which has no corresponding thallium uptake and was attributable to an intrathyroidal cyst. (**C**) The subtraction image shows the excess thallium uptake beneath the left lower thyroid lobe (*arrow*), caused by a parathyroid adenoma.

nique. In this case, the area of excess thallium accumulation is obvious without subtraction.

ADRENAL CORTICAL UPTAKE AND IMAGING

Cholesterol, chiefly from the blood, is the precursor for adreno-cortical synthesis of adrenal hormones through a pregnenolone intermediary compound. Glucocorticoid synthesis is controlled via the pituitary servomechanism for ACTH secretion, which in turn is regulated by corticotropin-releasing hormone from the hypothalamus. Abnormal secretion of adrenal glucocorticoids may be due to abnormal secretion of pituitary ACTH or ectopic production of ACTH, leading to adrenal cortical hyperplasia, or benign or malignant tumors arising from the adrenal cortex. Hypersecretion of the mineral corticoid, aldosterone, may be due to nodular adrenal hyperplasia or benign or malignant adrenal cortical neoplasms. The diagnosis of these conditions must be established biochemically using appropriate measurements of serum hormone levels and monitoring these levels in response to adrenal suppression maneuvers. Urinary measurements of ster-oid production and metabolism reflect a more long-term estimate of adrenocortical function, as does adrenal uptake of radiolabeled cholesterol. Once the diagnosis of adrenocortical hyperfunction has been made, determination of the cause and localization of a neoplasm, if present, is the next step.

Adrenal uptake of the cholesterol analogue, ^{131}I-labeled norcholesterol, NP-59, can provide corroboration of adrenocor-tical hyperfunction, especially when used with appropriate sup-pressive maneuvers. Expansion of the cholesterol-carrying pool of chylomicrons and low-density lipoproteins (LDLs) as well as various drugs such as oral contraceptives and diuretics and changes in the patient's electrolyte status can affect the re-sults.

The major diagnostic benefit of adrenocortical imaging with ^{131}I-labeled norcholesterol is localizing neoplasms that can be surgically removed, leading to cure. This is particularly helpful in the patient with a suspected adrenal remnant following previous surgical curative attempts. Symmetric increased uptake indicates ACTH-dependent hyperplasia, while marked asymmetry indicates hypercorticalism independent of ACTH secretion. Unilateral visualization suggests a unilateral neoplasm, usually an adenoma, suppressing the normal nonvisualized adrenal gland. Nonvisualization of functioning adrenal tissue on the scan in cases in which technical causes for this have been excluded is consistent with the presence of a functioning adrenocortical carcinoma, bulky enough to produce sufficient hormone to suppress the normal contralateral gland but having insufficient uptake per unit volume to permit visualization. Alternatively, the adrenocortical carcinoma may cause nonvisualization of the affected adrenal gland because of destructive replacement of normal adrenal tissue.

In distinguishing between ACTH-induced adrenal hyperplasia and primary adrenal tumors that produce hypercortisolism, radionuclide adrenocortical imaging has produced very accurate results. Results have been helpful but not as reliable in Conn's syndrome of hyperaldosteronism. Reports have suggested the value of this technique in distinguishing between adrenal and ovarian causes of hirsutism. Unfortunately, this scanning technique remains investigational and is limited to a few university medical centers in the United States, despite the elapse of 17 years since its introduction as a clinically useful technique. Nonetheless, when purely biochemical techniques and anatomic investigations such as computed tomography (CT) or magnetic resonance imaging (MRI) do not produce clear-cut answers, this elegant means of imaging the physiology of steroid synthesis should be used. Figure 3-5 shows a norcholesterol image in a man with Cushing's disease, bilateral adrenal hyperplasia resulting from a pituitary adenoma producing excess ACTH. Symmetric increased activity is apparent in the adrenal glands; a renal scan performed immediately following the ^{131}I NP-59 imaging without moving the patient confirms the adrenal location of the radiolabeled norcholesterol activity.

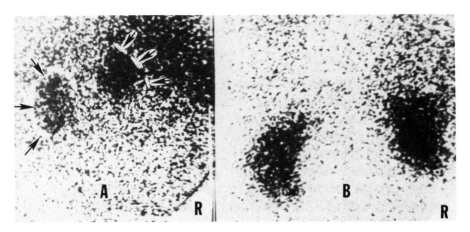

FIG. 3-5. Adrenal cortical hyperplasia due to pituitary adenoma (Cushing's disease) with bilateral visualization of the adrenal glands (*arrows*) in spite of dexamethasone suppression. (**A**) Norcholesterol scan shows clear-cut activity in both adrenal glands. (**B**) Renal image with ^{99m}Tc DTPA performed without moving the patient following the norcholesterol image shows the relationship of the norcholesterol uptake to the kidneys, indicating that the norcholesterol uptake is in the normal adrenal sites.

ADRENAL MEDULLARY IMAGING

A similar approach used to localize adrenal medullary neoplasms has also found application in diagnosis and treatment of neural crest-derivative neoplasms, so-called APUD neoplasms. The norepinephrine and guanethidine analogue, ^{131}I-labeled metaiodobenzylguanidine ($[^{131}I]$MIBG), is taken up at sites of catecholamine storage granules. Thus, sites of synthesis of excess catecholamines may be detected by imaging the distribution of $[^{131}I]$MIBG. This has proved accurate in localizing adrenal pheochromocytomas, extra-adrenal (paraganglionoma) tumor sites, adrenal medullary hyperplasia, and certain neoplasms such as neuroblastoma, carcinoid, and medullary thyroid carcinomas.

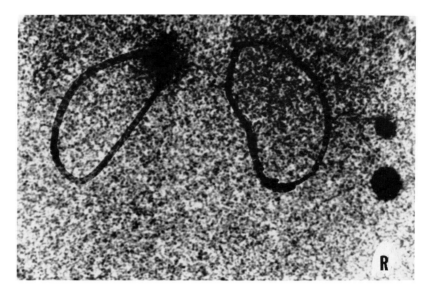

FIG. 3-6. Left adrenal pheochromocytoma visualized with $[^{131}I]$MIBG in a 28-yr-old man with a history of dizzy spells and one episode of syncope. The blood pressure measured 218/70 mm Hg. The abnormal uptake can be seen to be localized in the left adrenal area from the superimposed tracing of the kidney outlines obtained by performing a renal image with ^{99m}Tc DTPA without moving the patient after the MIBG scan. (Case courtesy of Azzizullah Ansari, M.D., USC/LAC Medical Center, Los Angeles.)

Figure 3-6 shows a left adrenal pheochromocytoma. Functional neoplasm imaging with MIBG remains restricted to investigative centers in the United States, but initial results suggest that it can be helpful when purely anatomic results from CT imaging remain uncertain or even misleading. The ability to detect functioning tissue remains unique, and the promise this holds for therapeutic application is being investigated. The high target uptake of MIBG makes it possible to deliver high doses of radiation to functioning primary and metastatic neoplasms that concentrate $[^{131}I]$MIBG.

SELECTED READINGS

Thyroid Function

Hamburger JI. Application of the radioiodine uptake to the clinical evaluation of thyroid disease. *Semin Nucl Med* 1971; 1: 287–300

Werner SC, Ingbar SH (eds). *The thyroid: A fundamental and clinical text.* 2nd ed. Hagerstown, MD: Harper & Row; 1978

Thyroid Imaging

Charkes ND. Scintigraphic evaluation of nodular goiter. *Semin Nucl Med* 1971; 1:316–333

dos Remedios LV, Weber PM, Jasko IA. Thyroid scintigraphy in 1000 patients: Rational use of Tc-99m and I-131 compounds. *J Nucl Med* 1971; 12:673–677

Pinsky S, Ryo UY. Thyroid imaging: A current status report. In: Freeman LM, Weissmann HS, eds. *Nuclear medicine annual 1981.* New York: Raven Press; 1981:157–194

Thyroid Carcinoma

Hurley JR, Becker DV. The use of radioiodine in the management of thyroid cancer. In: Freeman LM and Weissmann HS, eds. *Nuclear medicine annual 1983.* New York: Raven Press; 1983: 329–384

Mazzaferri EL, Young RL. Papillary thyroid carcinoma: A 10-year follow-up report of the impact of therapy in 576 patients. *Am J Med* 1981; 70:511–518

Parathyroid Imaging

Winzelberg GG. Parathyroid imaging. *Ann Intern Med* 1987; 107: 64–70

Young AE, Gaunt JI, Croft DN, et al. Localization of parathyroid adenomas by thallium-201 and technetium-99m subtraction scanning. *Br Med J* 1983; 286:1384–1386

Adrenocortical Imaging

Guerin CK, Wahner HW, Gorman CA, et al. Computed tomographic scanning versus radioisotope imaging in adrenocortical diagnosis. *Am J Med* 1983; 75:653–657

Hogan MJ, McCrae J, Schambelan M, Biglieri EG. Location of aldosterone-producing adenomas with [131]I-19-iodocholesterol. *N Engl J Med* 1976; 294:410–414

Lieberman LM, Beierwaltes WH, Conn JW, et al. Diagnosis of adrenal disease by visualization of human adrenal glands with [131]I-19-iodocholesterol. *N Engl J Med* 1971; 285:1387–1393

Adrenergic Tumor Imaging and Therapy

Hoefnagel CA, Vout PA, de Kraker J, Marcuse HR. Radionuclide diagnosis and therapy of neural crest tumors using iodine-131 metaiodobenzylguanidine. *J Nucl Med* 1987; 28:308–314

McEwan AJ, Shapiro B, Sisson JC, et al. Radio-iodobenzylguanidine for the scintigraphic location and therapy of adrenergic tumors. *Semin Nucl Med* 1985; 15:132–153

Sisson JC, Frager M, Valk T, et al. Scintigraphic localization of pheochromocytoma. *N Engl J Med* 1981; 305:12–17

Von Moll L, McEwan AJ, Shapiro B, et al. Iodine—131 MIBG scintigraphy of neuroendocrine tumors other than pheochromoytoma and neuroblastoma. *J Nucl Med* 1987; 28:979–988

4

Cardiovascular System

Nuclear medicine imaging and data processing techniques provide accurate, repeatable evaluation of cardiac structure, perfusion, and function. These approaches have application in patients with coronary artery disease, congenital and valvular heart disease, and cardiomyopathy.

CARDIAC BLOOD-POOL IMAGING AND EVALUATION OF VENTRICULAR FUNCTION

Radioisotopic imaging of the cardiac blood pool is performed after intravenous (i.v.) injection of a radiopharmaceutical, such as ^{99m}Tc-labeled red cells, which remains in the intravascular space. In vivo, "in vivtro," and in vitro techniques for labeling red cells are used.*

Gated images of the labeled cardiac blood pool (MUGA study) evaluate left ventricular function and regional ventricular wall motion. These images are obtained by gating, or triggering, the scintillation camera's count acquisitions to the electrocardiogram (ECG) signal. Images of the heart in systole and diastole are created by summing counts obtained during end-systole and end-diastole over many cardiac cycles. Images of other short intervals throughout the cardiac cycle may be obtained as well. The cardiac cycle can be subdivided into 16–64 frames; counts for each frame are accumulated from many heart beats to form the multiple images of a composite heart beat. This collection of

---

*"In vivtro" designates a combined in vivo–in vitro technique.

counts requires a stable, regular rhythm. In patients with arrhythmias, the use of computer programs designed to eliminate "bad beats" is necessary. The resulting images from each portion of the cardiac cycle can be viewed individually or, more importantly, can be displayed in cinematic fashion on the computer video display as a motion picture of the beating heart. The perception of regional wall motion abnormalities is greatly improved by this cinematic display format. In the left anterior oblique projection, the left ventricle can be visualized without overlap from the other cardiac chambers (Fig. 4-1A). The counts detected in the left ventricle are proportional to volume, and the change from end-systolic counts (ESC) to end-diastolic counts (EDC) of the left ventricle can be used for the calculation of left ventricular ejection fraction from the formula:

$$\text{Ejection fraction} = \frac{\text{EDC} - \text{ESC}}{\text{EDC}}.$$

The left ventricular ejection fraction is a sensitive indicator of left ventricular dysfunction. The ejection fraction is normally >50%; however, patients with recent myocardial infarction show a decrease in ejection fraction that is closely correlated with the volume of infarcted myocardium, as well as with prognosis.

Serial measurements of left ventricular ejection fraction are likely to assume increasing importance in the management of patients with myocardial infarction as more vigorous therapeutic interventions designed to protect ischemic myocardium are employed in these patients. Under these circumstances, ejection fraction measurements can be helpful in determining whether a patient is suitable for a particular type of intervention. These measurements may also be used to indicate whether therapy is significantly improving or adversely affecting left ventricular performance. This application has been greatly facilitated by the development of mobile scintillation cameras and computers. Thus, gated cardiac imaging, as well as many other nuclear medicine studies, may be performed at the bedside of critically ill patients in intensive care units.

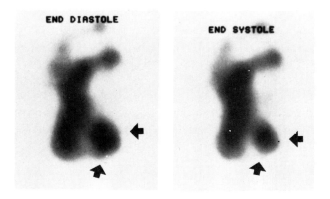

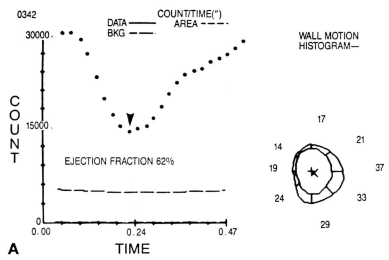

FIG. 4-1. (A) Normal patient: Left anterior oblique views of end-diastole and end-systole obtained using ^{99m}Tc-labeled autologous red blood cells show good wall motion of the left ventricle (*arrows*). In this view, the interventricular septum is seen clearly as a region of decreased counts between the left ventricle and the right ventricle. The lower left panel shows computer printout of ejection fraction, 62% in this normal patient, and the volume curve of left ventricular counts versus time for a composite r-to-r interval (cardiac cycle). The lower right panel shows the contours of end-diastole (*outer circle*) and end-systole (*inner circle*) super-imposed. Good wall motion between diastole and systole is seen. The high septal region, corresponding to numbers 14–19 on the wall-motion display, is a region of valve planes and therefore cannot be analyzed for wall motion.

55

Gated cardiac blood-pool images have also shown high sensitivity in detecting regional left ventricular wall motion abnormalities. Regions of hypokinesis, akinesis, or dyskinesis (paradoxical wall motion, as with a left ventricular aneurysm) are found in most patients with myocardial infarction (Fig. 4-1B).

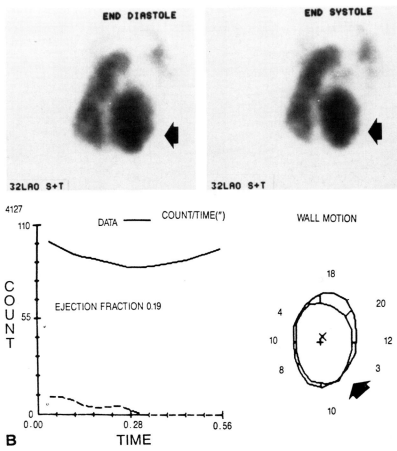

FIG. 4-1. (B) Abnormal patient: The gated blood-pool images at end-diastole and end-systole show generalized severe left ventricular hypokinesis (*arrows*). The calculated ejection fraction is 19%; the contour images of end-diastole and end-systole (*lower right panel*) show akinesis in the posterior inferior wall (*arrow*).

The size of the ventricular region exhibiting abnormal wall motion also correlates closely with the size of the myocardial infarct. In patients with congestive cardiac failure, evaluation of ventricular wall motion can be useful in distinguishing patients with global ventricular dysfunction from those with segmental abnormalities who might respond to corrective surgical intervention.

Cinematic cardiac blood-pool images may be obtained in patients at rest and during bicycle exercise. In patients with coronary artery disease in whom focal ischemia develops during exercise, the exercise images may demonstrate new regional wall motion abnormalities. Furthermore, the left ventricular ejection fraction usually falls or remains unchanged during exercise in patients with coronary artery disease, whereas it increases substantially in normal subjects. Thus, this technique appears to be a simple means of detecting stress-induced myocardial ischemia with a sensitivity of 87–95% and similar specificity in selected populations. Caution, however, is important in interpreting this test, since some patients may fail to achieve exercise levels adequate to stress the heart, causing false-negative results. Some normal populations, notably women, are known to fail to show a consistent normal ejection fraction response to exercise. Other diseases that affect myocardial function, such as cardiomyopathy and valvular disease, may give abnormal ejection fraction response to stress as well.

Additional information obtained from gated cardiac blood-pool studies includes (1) right ventricular ejection fraction, (2) count-derived estimates of ventricular volumes, and (3) regurgitant fraction in patients with valvular heart disease. Other applications of the technique include (1) evaluation of the response to exercise in asymptomatic patients with valvular heart disease to permit improved timing of valve replacement surgery; (2) earlier and more reliable detection of Adriamycin-induced cardiotoxicity, permitting greater individualization of the course of chemotherapy with this drug; and (3) evaluation of right ventricular and left ventricular function in patients with obstructive lung disease.

RADIONUCLIDE ANGIOCARDIOGRAPHY

Radionuclide angiocardiography is performed by rapid i.v. injection of a radioactive bolus followed by sequential imaging with the scintillation camera to record its passage through the circulation. Technetium-99m sodium pertechnetate or ^{99m}Tc labeled to any of a number of compounds in a 370–925 MBq (10–25 mCi) dose is employed for this purpose. Dose variations depend on collimation, patient size, and instrumentation.

Evaluation of ventricular function can be performed with radionuclide angiocardiography as well as with the gated cardiac imaging techniques described earlier. For this purpose, the radionuclide angiocardiogram is recorded by computer, and the time–activity curve is generated from a region of interest placed over the region of the left ventricle and is subsequently displayed. The high-frequency data from the angiocardiogram demonstrate the beat-to-beat oscillations in ventricular activity, which correspond to changes in ventricular volume. This permits calculation of left and right ventricular ejection fractions.

Radionuclide angiocardiography measures the transit of a bolus through the central circulation. These data, like dye dilution curves, may be used as a screening procedure in patients with suspected congenital heart disease. Gross anatomic aberrations can often be identified on the images, which are obtained after a peripheral intravenous injection. In cases in which clinical differentiation of left-to-right shunt lesions from functional murmurs is difficult, this procedure or echocardiography may obviate the need for cardiac catheterization. Similarly, in cyanotic infants, right-to-left shunts can be diagnosed and differentiated from other causes of cyanosis. The normal angiocardiogram demonstrates serial appearance of the radionuclide bolus in the cardiac chambers in normal sequence without evidence of chamber dilatation, delay in transit, or rapid recirculation.

A left-to-right shunt can be detected by the rapid recirculation of tracer to the lungs once it enters the left side of the heart. Using a dedicated computer system, prolongation of the transit in the right side of the circulation may also be detected by quantitative analysis of the time–activity curve over the lung, which will permit shunts as small as 10% to be diagnosed and quantitated from the calculated pulmonic : systemic flow ratio. Cardiac function of patients with small ventricular septal defects can be evaluated by repeated radionuclide angiocardiograms to confirm that the shunt is closing spontaneously. Similarly, the radionuclide study is useful in evaluating the adequacy of corrective surgery.

Radionuclide angiocardiography indicates an intracardiac right-to-left shunt by the appearance of the bolus in the left side of the heart and aorta before the appearance of lung activity. Whereas it is frequently possible to ascertain the level of the shunt, this technique is by no means as accurate as standard radiographic angiocardiography in delineating the anatomy of the lesion.

Radionuclide angiography can also be employed as a rapid screening procedure in diagnosing major vascular obstructive lesions. Obstruction of the superior vena cava or of the abdominal aorta is readily diagnosed with this technique. Peripheral vascular obstruction may also be detected.

EVALUATION OF MYOCARDIAL PERFUSION

Thallium-201 (^{201}Tl) chloride is treated similarly to potassium by myocardial cells. Both thallium and potassium need the Na^+/K^+—ATPase pump for active transport into cells. Regional myocardial uptake of ^{201}Tl reflects myocardial blood supply, myocardial cell viability, and integrity of membrane sodium–potassium transport systems. Myocardial uptake and blood clearance of this radiopharmaceutical are rapid, and imaging can be started 5–10 min after intravenous injection, or immediately for stress thallium studies. The normal myocardial perfusion image shows uniform distribution of activity in the left ventricular myocardium, with the ventricular cavity appearing as a central region of decreased counts in the image. For complete evaluation of myocardial perfusion, multiple images are obtained in several projections or single-photon emission computed tomography (SPECT) may be performed.

Regions of myocardial ischemia or infarct appear on ^{201}Tl chloride images as focal areas of diminished activity. Thus, on the basis of a single ^{201}Tl chloride imaging study alone, it is not possible to distinguish transient myocardial ischemia, acute myocardial infarction, or myocardial scar from prior infarction. Approximately 90% of patients with acute transmural myocardial infarction will have abnormal ^{201}Tl chloride scans if imaged within 24 hr postinfarction. Nontransmural infarcts are more difficult to detect. The experience in quantitating myocardial infarct size from ^{201}Tl chloride images has been variable.

A more important application of ^{201}Tl chloride imaging is in the diagnosis of transient myocardial ischemia. For this purpose, the thallium images are combined with a conventional exercise stress test. The ^{201}Tl chloride is injected intravenously toward the end of the exercise stress test. When stress images are compared with baseline rest or later redistribution images, new perfusion defects indicate the presence of focal, exercise-induced myocardial ischemia. These scintigraphic findings correlate well with the findings of high-grade coronary artery stenosis by coronary angiography. As an alternative to obtaining separate resting and postexercise studies, delayed imaging is performed at most laboratories 3–5 hr after the initial stress images. During this interval, ^{201}Tl is redistributed to zones of the left ventricle that were transiently ischemic during exercise, whereas zones of infarction do not change in appearance (Fig. 4-2). Focal exercise-induced perfusion defects are found in 73–95% of patients with angiographically significant coronary artery disease, whereas the conventional exercise ECG will be abnormal in only ~60% of cases. False-negative studies may result from the presence of small zones of ischemia that cannot be resolved on thallium images or from severe three-vessel coronary artery disease in which global, but not focal, ischemia may be present. This latter problem, although not frequent, emphasizes the fact that

Stress

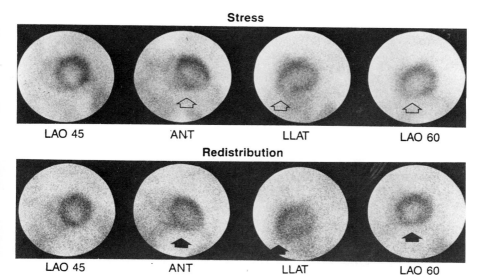

LAO 45   ANT   LLAT   LAO 60

Redistribution

LAO 45   ANT   LLAT   LAO 60

FIG. 4-2. Myocardial perfusion imaging with ^{201}Tl during stress and redistribution: Multiple planar views at stress show a region of impaired perfusion (*open arrows*) in the inferoapical wall of the left ventricle. At redistribution, 4 hr later (*lower panel*), the images show thallium activity in the inferoapical left ventricular wall (*black arrows*) indicating ischemia rather than myocardial scar.

myocardial perfusion images reflect relative myocardial perfusion, but not absolute blood flow.

Other applications of ^{201}Tl imaging include differentiation of ischemic and idiopathic cardiomyopathy, evaluation of the functional significance of collateral coronary vessels seen at angiography, evaluating efficacy of percutaneous transluminal angioplasty in coronary artery stenosis, and assessment of the patency of coronary artery bypass grafts. Thallium-201 chloride images also show right ventricular hypertrophy, if present. Under normal circumstances, only the left ventricular myocardium is well visualized at rest. With right ventricular hypertrophy, uptake of thallium in the wall of the right ventricle becomes increasingly prominent. Similarly, in patients with asymmetric septal hypertrophy, the ^{201}Tl chloride images may permit direct assessment of septal thickness. Computer programs to analyze quantitatively the relative perfusion and washout in regions of the left ventricular myocardium at rest and exercise have been devised to aid in thallium image interpretations. At centers where SPECT is available, tomographic images of myocardial thallium uptake have been found very useful (Fig. 4-3), with reports of 10–25% increased sensitivity over planar imaging.

The recent introduction of ^{99m}Tc isonitrile compounds promises to provide a more readily available, cheaper radiopharmaceutical that will enhance the quality of myocardial perfusion

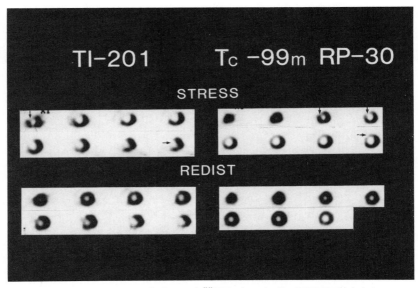

FIG. 4-3. Thallium-201 (left) and ^{99m}Tc isonitrile SPECT (right) stress and redistribution (rest) images in a patient with ischemia of the anteroseptal wall of the left ventricle. Transverse cross-sectional images (short–axis views) of the left ventricle are shown: Thallium-201 images with injection during stress show anteroseptal perfusion deficiency on the tomographic slices from just above the apex (↓) to base (→) of the left ventricle. Technetium-99m isonitrile images (^{99m}Tc RP-30) also show anteroseptal perfusion deficit from just above the apex (↓) to the base (→). Redistribution thallium and rest ^{99m}Tc isonitrile images show that thallium nearly completely fills in the anteroseptal deficit seen at stress and ^{99m}Tc isonitrile images show a normal perfusion pattern.

imaging, particularly with SPECT. Unlike thallium, these compounds do not redistribute into ischemic areas with time. Using thallium, differentiation of exercise-induced ischemia from infarction depends on imaging the redistribution of thallium into ischemic regions over a 3–4-hr period. With thallium, imaging must be performed immediately following an injection made during maximal exercise and after a 3–4-hr or longer delay or a separate injection of thallium made with the patient at rest. The new ^{99m}Tc isonitrile compounds eliminate dependence on redistribution to establish the diagnosis of ischemia. The exercise study is performed following injection of the ^{99m}Tc isonitrile made during peak exercise. The rest distribution image uses a second injection made with the patient resting. The use of different doses for exercise and rest studies may permit completion of the study at a single session. The resulting SPECT images, because of higher count rates and the more favorable energy emission of ^{99m}Tc over ^{201}Tl, are superior and less subject to attenuation artifacts commonly seen with ^{201}Tl. Figure 4-3 shows an exercise and a rest study performed with ^{99m}Tc-labeled isonitrile demonstrating ischemic myocardial disease, compared with a stress and redistribution thallium study in the same patient. Ready availability, decreased cost, increased count rate permitting a shorter imaging time and increased image quality, and decreased radiation dose as compared with thallium favor the use of a ^{99m}Tc-labeled agent. In addition, the high photon yield from the ^{99m}Tc-labeled agent permits performance of a first-pass dynamic cardiac study if imaging over the cardiac region is done at the time of i.v. bolus injection. Such a study also yields information concerning cardiac wall motion and provides data for cardiac ejection fraction calculation.

PET IMAGING, BLOOD FLOW AND METABOLISM

Although not yet available on a routine clinical basis, PET imaging (see discussion of PET imaging in Chapter 1, page 16) can depict regional myocardial blood flow using ^{13}N labeled ammonia or ^{82}Rb and regional myocardial metabolism using ^{18}F fluorodeoxyglucose and labeled fatty acids. The normal myocardium preferentially uses fatty acid metabolism. Ischemic but viable myocardium increases glucose utilization, which has a lower oxygen requirement than fat metabolism. PET imaging shows that ischemic myocardium has a relative decrease in fatty acid uptake, a relative increase in deoxyglucose uptake, and a relative reduction in perfusion. Figure 4-4 shows PET images of perfusion/metabolic mismatches in ischemic myocardium.

MYOCARDIAL INFARCT IMAGING

Although a variety of radiopharmaceuticals have been shown to localize in zones of recent myocardial necrosis, the most widely used agent is ^{99m}Tc pyrophosphate, a bone-seeking radiophar-

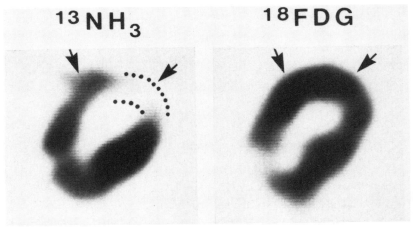

FIG. 4-4. Ischemic myocardium indicated by PET imaging of sections through the mid-left ventricle. The image on the left with ^{13}N ammonia depicting myocardial perfusion shows a defect in the anterior septum and anterior wall (*arrows*). The image on the right with ^{18}F fluorodeoxyglucose shows uptake of exogenous glucose by this same region. This mismatch indicates ischemic, but viable myocardium. (Case courtesy of Heinrich R. Schelbert, M.D., Professor of Radiological Sciences, UCLA Center for the Health Sciences, Los Angeles, California.) (Reproduced by permission from *J Mol Cell Cardiol* 1984; 16:683–93.)

maceutical (Fig. 4-5). The precise mechanism of uptake of these agents in regions of necrosis is unknown. However, it is presumed that they bind to intracellular deposits of inorganic calcium salts, which form in dying myocardial cells. Uptake of pyrophosphate indicates active myocytolysis and other causes of phosphate deposition.

Imaging is performed 2–3 hr after i.v. injection of 370–555 MBq (10–15 mCi) of ^{99m}Tc pyrophosphate. Positive uptake of the radiopharmaceutical occurs in regions of damaged myocardium as early as 12 hr postinfarction. Peak intensity of tracer accumulation occurs 48–72 hr after infarction and, in most cases, no abnormality will be apparent after 10 days. However, in ~30% of patients, myocardial infarction images will remain abnormal indefinitely after transmural infarction, particularly in those in whom left ventricular aneurysms develop. Transmural infarction is detected with >90% sensitivity and can usually be accurately localized by evaluation of anterior, lateral, and oblique views.

This test is less accurate in diagnosing subendocardial myocardial infarction. In these cases, a positive test often demonstrates diffuse myocardial uptake rather than focal accumulation. False-positive images can result from slow blood-

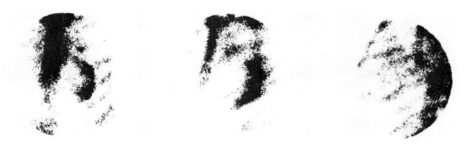

Anterior   LAO   Left Lateral

FIG. 4-5. Anterior, left anterior oblique (LAO), and left lateral views of a ^{99m}Tc pyrophosphate scan in a patient who suffered a transmural myocardial infarct ~2 days before the scan. Normal rib and sternum uptake are seen, as well as abnormal uptake in the posterolateral myocardium.

pool clearance of the radiopharmaceutical, although a 24-hr delayed image will usually show resolution of the activity unless a true acute myocardial infarct is present.

Single-photon emission computed tomography has also been shown to contribute to the true-positive identification of focal acute infarcts in patients in whom planar images were equivocal. In addition to acute infarction, abnormal scans have been observed resulting from the myocytolysis that accompanies unstable angina pectoris, cardiomyopathy, and cardioversion as well as amyloidosis.

Another experimental approach to imaging acute myocardial infarction that appears to have increased specificity is a labeled antibody technique using labeled antimyosin Fab fragments.

SELECTED READINGS

General

Berman DS, Mason DT (eds). *Clinical nuclear cardiology.* New York: Grune & Stratton; 1981

Holman BL. Radioisotopic examination of the cardiovascular system. In: Braunwald E, ed. *Heart disease: A textbook of cardiovascular medicine.* 2nd ed. Philadelphia: WB Saunders; 1984: 351–400

Iskandrian AS. *Nuclear cardiac imaging: Principles and applications,* Philadelphia: FA Davis Co; 1987

Rozanski A, Berman D. Efficacy of cardiovascular nuclear medicine studies. *Semin Nucl Med* 1987; 17:104–120

Strauss HW, Pitt B (eds). *Cardiovascular nuclear medicine.* 2nd ed. St Louis: CV Mosby; 1979

Cardiac Blood-Pool Imaging

Borer JS, Bachrach SL, Green MV, et al. Rapid evaluation of left ventricular function during exercise in patients with coronary artery disease. *N Engl J Med* 1977; 296:839–844

Strauss HW, Zaret BL, Hurley PJ, et al. A scintiphotographic method for measuring left ventricular ejection fraction in man without cardiac catheterization. *Am J Cardiol* 1971; 28:575–580

Radionuclide Angiocardiography

Schelbert HR, Henning H, Asburn WL, et al. Serial measurement of left ventricular ejection fraction by radionuclide angiography early and late after myocardial infarction. *Am J Cardiol* 1976; 38:407–415

Treves S, Maltz DL. Radionuclide angiocardiography. *Postgrad Med J* 1974; 56:99–107

Weber PM, dos Remedios LV, Jasko IA. Quantitative radioisotope angiocardiography. *J Nucl Med* 1972; 13:815–822

Evaluation of Myocardial Perfusion

Alderson PO, Coleman RE, Grove RB, et al (eds). *Nuclear radiology (Third Series) syllabus*. Chicago: American College of Radiology; 1983:87–90, 104–117

Berman DS, Garcia EV, Maddahi J. Role of thallium-201 imaging in the diagnosis of myocardial ischemia and infarction. In: Freeman LM, Weissmann HS, eds. *Nuclear medicine annual 1980*. New York: Raven Press; 1980:1–55

Marshall RC, Tillisch JH, Phelps ME, et al. Identification and differentiation of resting myocardial ischemia and infarction in man with positron computed tomography ^{18}F-labeled fluoro-deoxyglucose and N-13 ammonia. *Circulation* 1981; 64: 766–778, 1981

McKillop JH. Thallium-201 scintigraphy. *West J Med* 1980; 133:26–43

McKusick KA, Holman BL, Rigo P, et al. Human myocardial imaging with 99m Tc isonitriles (abstract). *Circulation* 1986; 74:II–296

Myocardial Infarct Imaging

Khaw BA, Gold HK, Yasuda T, et al. Scintigraphic quantification of myocardial necrosis in patients after intravenous injection of myosin-specific antibody. *Circulation* 1986; 74:501–508

Poliner LR, Buja LM, Parkey RW, et al. Clinicopathologic findings in 52 patients studied by technetium 99m stannous pyrophosphate myocardial scintigraphy. *Circulation* 1979; 59:257–267

5

Pulmonary System and Thromboembolism

DIAGNOSIS OF PULMONARY EMBOLISM

Pulmonary embolism continues to be a major health problem, with considerable controversy surrounding the diagnostic approaches and their interpretation. The magnitude of the problem has been summarized by Dalen and Alpert, who estimate that 600,000 patients have clinically significant pulmonary embolism and that 120,000 die annually from this disease in the United States without being diagnosed.

The problems in diagnosis of pulmonary embolism relate to the nonspecificity of clinical signs and symptoms and to the relatively invasive nature and high financial costs associated with the definitive diagnostic procedure of pulmonary angiography. The radionuclide lung scan is a highly sensitive test for diagnosis of pulmonary embolism; it is widely used because it is safe, readily available, easily performed, and provides clinically important information.

Most pulmonary medicine physicians, angiographers, and nuclear medicine physicians would agree that (1) a normal perfusion scan indicates no major emboli; (2) an abnormal perfusion scan alone is a nonspecific indicator of emboli, but a perfusion/ventilation study showing mismatched abnormalities indicates high probability of primary pulmonary vascular disease such as pulmonary emboli; and (3) the perfusion scan guides the selection of sites for angiography.

PRINCIPLES OF PULMONARY PERFUSION/ VENTILATION IMAGING

The radionuclide pulmonary perfusion imaging study records relative regional pulmonary arterial blood flow. It is based on the principle of capillary blockade. Particles larger than the size of the smallest capillaries are trapped in the first capillary bed they reach after peripheral intravenous injection. Labeled particles ~20–40 μm in size are injected intravenously and trapped in the capillary bed of the lungs. The labeled particles are assumed to be well mixed in the blood after passage through the right atrium and ventricle; thus, their distribution in the lung capillaries truly reflects the distribution of pulmonary artery blood flow in the lungs.

The most widely used radiopharmaceuticals are ^{99m}Tc labeled to albumin microspheres or ^{99m}Tc labeled to macroaggregates of albumin. Radiation exposure is in the range of 3×10^{-5}–10^{-4} Gy/MBq (0.1–0.4 rad/mCi) of ^{99m}Tc particles to the critical organ, the lungs. Most adult doses are in the range of 74–148 MBq (2–4 mCi). A xenon-133 (^{133}Xe) ventilation lung scan usually gives < 0.01 Gy (1 rad) to the lungs and about 0.03–0.04 Gy (3–4 rad) to the mucosa of the tracheobronchial tree, depending on dose and technique.

Approximately 100,000–500,000 particles are injected with an adult dose of ^{99m}Tc-labeled particles for perfusion lung imaging. Estimates suggest that there are 280 billion capillaries in the lungs. Therefore, the safety factor in percentage of capillaries embolized by the labeled particles is many orders of magnitude, making the procedure safe. In patients with severe pulmonary disease, particularly pulmonary hypertension, it may be prudent to inject no more than 100,000 particles. The particles are broken down in the lungs by macrophage activity and physical and enzymatic processes, so that their biologic half-life in the lungs is ~5–12 hr.

Images of the distribution of the labeled particles show focal regions of decreased activity where there is diminished pulmonary artery blood flow, as occurs distal to the site of an embolus. Many other pathologic processes, including pneumonia, emphysema, tumor, atelectasis, and almost any process that reduces regional ventilation, diminish pulmonary arterial blood flow as well. Therefore, lung scans cannot be accurately interpreted without a current x-ray film of the chest (within hours of the scan) and knowledge of regional ventilation.

VENTILATION IMAGING

Ventilation images describe the regional patterns of washin and washout of materials inspired in the lungs. Ventilation imaging may be performed using inert gases such as xenon-133 (^{133}Xe), ^{127}Xe, or ^{81m}Kr or an aerosol such as ^{99m}Tc DTPA. While the inert gases have the appeal of reflecting a truer physiologic representation of ventilatory function, a high degree of agreement has been documented for aerosol imaging as a reasonable, more easily performed and potentially less expensive alternative to standard gas ventilation imaging.

Xenon-133 gas is the most widely used agent for ventilation imaging. The standard procedure is to obtain images of the washin, equilibrium, and washout patterns from the lungs while the patient breathes the radioactive xenon gas mixed with air or oxygen, delivered via a mouthpiece from a spirometry gas delivery system. Alternatively, the ^{133}Xe gas can be given as a bolus, which the patient inspires. Ventilation imaging can also be performed using a radiolabeled aerosol delivered through a nebulizer. This technique permits imaging of inspiration only, since the aerosolized particles adhere to mucosal surfaces and are not washed out with expired air. Clearance rates from the lungs of aerosolized small-molecular-weight compounds, such as ^{99m}Tc DTPA, may be used as a measure of interstitial lung disease. Rapid clearance rates have been associated with disease.

SENSITIVITY OF PULMONARY PERFUSION IMAGING IN DETECTING PULMONARY EMBOLISM

In animal experiments, Moser et al. (1969) documented that pulmonary perfusion imaging and pulmonary angiography agree closely in detecting pulmonary emboli, although both tests miss some emboli. Alderson et al. (1978) demonstrated that selective pulmonary angiography is more sensitive than perfusion lung imaging for detecting small, peripheral emboli and emboli that partially obstruct pulmonary vessels. Nonetheless, their work demonstrated that radionuclide pulmonary perfusion imaging detected most emboli (87%) large enough to occlude vessels > 1 mm in diameter. In practice, however, since symptomatic patients apparently rarely have pulmonary emboli that are all < 1 mm in diameter, perfusion lung scanning has been shown to approach 100% sensitivity in detecting embolic disease in a given patient.

SPECIFICITY OF RADIONUCLIDE PULMONARY PERFUSION IMAGING

Although the lung perfusion scan is apparently very sensitive in detecting patients with pulmonary embolic disease, its specificity is low, since a wide variety of pathologic processes show perfusion abnormalities on the lung scan. Segmental perfusion defects are more likely to be caused by pulmonary embolism, but there is no doubt that chronic obstructive pulmonary disease can result in identical findings.

To improve the specificity of the lung perfusion scan, the ventilation scan is used. Alderson et al. (1981) demonstrated that ventilation imaging is most likely to be helpful in a given patient if existing airway disease involves < 50% of the lung field ($\leq$ three of six lung zones show ventilation abnormalities). When two or more segmental or larger regions of V/P or $\dot{V}/\dot{Q}$ (ventilation/perfusion) mismatch are present, a high probability for pulmonary embolism is interpreted.

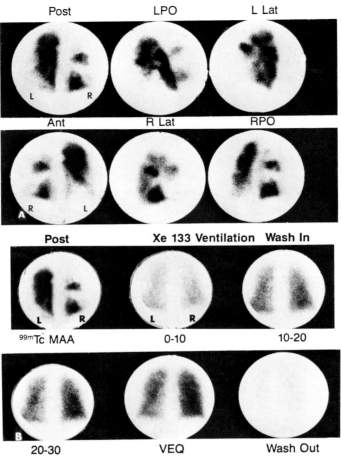

FIG. 5-1. (A) Perfusion lung scan performed after intravenous injection of ^{99m}Tc-labeled macroaggregates of albumin. Images in six projections taken over the lungs with the scintillation camera are shown. Multiple large segmental and lobar areas of abnormally diminished perfusion are shown to involve both lungs, particularly severely in the right lung. **(B)** Xenon-133 ventilation images are shown with the posterior view of the perfusion image in the upper far left panel. Washin phases of the ventilation are shown up to 30 sec, followed by the equilibrium image (*bottom middle*), followed by a single image of washout taken 2 min into the washout phase. The washin images show generally normal washin patterns in the right lung with some generalized diminished washin of the left lung. The regions of decreased perfusion in the right lung are mismatched with normal ventilation. The region of markedly decreased perfusion in the left lower lung field is also mismatched. The images suggest a high probability for pulmonary embolism in this patient.

72

Findings also suggest that a conservative approach to image interpretation is warranted in patients with extensive ventilation abnormalities. The high frequency of false-negative results in patients whose ventilation abnormalities involve more than 50% of the lung fields suggests that a nondiagnostic or indeterminate interpretation is appropriate. Theoretically, perfusion abnormalities in regions of lung that ventilate normally (V/P mismatch) indicate primary pulmonary vascular disease, such as pulmonary emboli (Fig. 5-1). Perfusion abnormalities associated with abnormal ventilation patterns (V/P match) reflect primary pulmonary parenchymal or airways disease (Fig. 5-2).

When pulmonary embolism results in infarction and a density on the chest film, the infarcted lung will not be normally ventilated. This abnormality may appear like any other parenchymal lung disease, showing corresponding ventilation and perfusion abnormalities. Using multiple matching projections—anterior, posterior, lateral, and oblique—of perfusion and aerosol imaging may permit more accurate anatomic delineation than possible with a single projection xenon ventilation image. Figure 5-3 shows selected views from perfusion and aerosol studies in a patient with pulmonary embolism and infarction. There are both V/P mismatches in the areas of embolism as well as V/P-matching defects in the area of infarction.

McNeil (1976) has demonstrated, in her review of ventilation/perfusion imaging and pulmonary angiography in 100 patients, a 100% sensitivity for the mismatched V/P scans in detecting pulmonary embolism. But, even the V/P mismatch is nonspecific for pulmonary thromboembolism. Ventilation/perfusion mismatch can be seen in primary pulmonary vascular diseases of other types, that is, pulmonary vasculitis, thrombosis in sickle cell disease, emboli other than thromboemboli (air, fat, tumor), mitral valve disease, and postradiation therapy (probably secondary to vasculitis).

Most physicians working in this field agree that when the radionuclide perfusion scan is normal, clinically significant pulmonary embolism can probably be ruled out. An abnormal perfusion scan and matched abnormal ventilation scan, although

Post   **Xe 133 Ventilation**

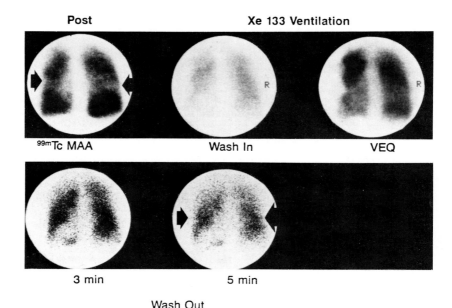

⁹⁹ᵐTc MAA   Wash In   VEQ

3 min   5 min

Wash Out

FIG. 5-2. Ventilation and perfusion images in the posterior projection show matching ventilation and perfusion abnormalities. There is marked decreased perfusion (*upper row, far left*) involving the middle and upper lung fields bilaterally (*arrows*). Xenon-133 ventilation images of washin and equilibrium (*upper row*) show slow washin to the lower and middle lung fields. Late washout images at 3 and 5 min (*lower panel*) show extensive trapping of gas in the upper and middle lung fields, extending into the lower lung field on the right (*arrows*). This study shows widespread abnormal ventilation in nearly every portion of the lungs. Perfusion abnormalities, although not quite as extensive as the ventilation abnormalities, are also widespread and evident in regions with abnormal ventilation. If this patient is being evaluated for pulmonary embolism, the interpretation of this study would be that pulmonary embolus cannot be diagnosed or excluded in the presence of such extensive ventilatory and perfusion abnormalities, consistent with pulmonary parenchymal and airways disease. In other words, an indeterminate reading would be given for this study.

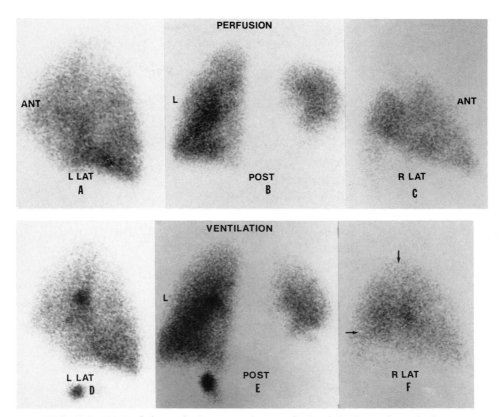

FIG. 5-3. (**A**) Left lateral, (**B**) posterior, and (**C**) right lateral perfusion images show a segmental perfusion defect of the right upper lobe apical segment as well as a lobar defect of the entire right lower lobe. The left lateral (**D**), posterior (**E**), and right lateral (**F**) views from the aerosol ventilation study show that the apical segment of the right upper lobe (vertical arrow) is normally ventilated and fills in with activity as does the superior segment of the right lower lobe (horizontal arrow). These V/P mismatches indicate vascular occlusive disease. The rest of the right lower lobe that had undergone infarction is not well ventilated, a V/P match indicating parenchymal lung disease, infarction in this case.

consistent with a primary pulmonary parenchymal or airways problem, cannot exclude a superimposed embolic phenomenon or embolism with infarction. Thus, a pulmonary angiogram must be performed in these indeterminate scan cases if a diagnosis of pulmonary embolic disease is to be confirmed or excluded. Finally, in the event of a V/P mismatch, the probability of pulmonary embolism is high, although other vascular abnormalities must be considered.

NONEMBOLIC PULMONARY DISEASE

Ventilation/perfusion imaging can be used to evaluate nonembolic pulmonary disorders, including restrictive lung disease, lung carcinoma, and obstructive airways disease. The V/P study can provide quantitative data on relative whole lung and regional lung function that may be useful to the surgeon in determining how much lung to resect and which regions are significant contributors to pulmonary function in patients with compromised pulmonary function. Using computer acquisitions, quantitative regional perfusion and ventilation are easily determined.

Peripheral intravenous injection of ^{133}Xe dissolved in saline may be used to measure relative regional lung perfusion, during arrival of activity in the lungs. Approximately 95% of the relatively insoluble xenon gas moves from the vascular space into the alveoli during the first passage through the pulmonary circulation. Subsequently, breathing removes the xenon from the lungs as any inert gas would be handled. A single injection can therefore quickly provide gross information concerning regional perfusion and ventilation. Such a technique can help clarify the pathophysiology of conditions that affect large areas of the lung, such as centrally located intrabronchial lesions, congenital lobar emphysema, the Swyer-James syndrome of unilateral hyperlucent lung, bullous lung disease, and lung injury from burns.

THROMBUS DETECTION

A variety of radionuclide techniques have been developed to detect arterial and venous thrombosis. At many institutions, radionuclide venography using ^{99m}Tc macroaggregated albumin is performed in conjunction with routine perfusion lung scanning. This technique detects obstruction of large veins. The deep venous system of the lower extremities is visualized by sequential

scintillation camera images after injection of a radiopharmaceutical into pedal veins with tourniquets tied proximally to
occlude superficial veins (Fig. 5-4). Deep-vein thrombosis is indicated by nonfilling of all or a portion of the deep venous
system, by filling of abnormal collateral vessels, or by the delayed
clearance of the particulate tracer from regions of venous stasis

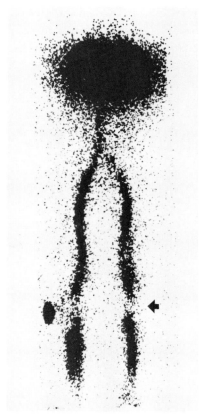

FIG. 5-4. Normal bilateral lower extremity venogram after ^{99m}Tc particle injection in veins in the feet of a patient referred for a lung scan. The
image shows single deep channels on each side. A spot and arrow mark
the popliteal fossa where tourniquets are in place to direct flow through
deep venous systems. The inverted wishbone appearance is formed by
the iliac veins uniting into the vena cava. Lungs are seen as very black
blob at top.

and at sites of venous endothelial injury (Fig. 5-5). For evaluation of large peripheral venous channels, radionuclide angiography with serial images after injection of a radionuclide such as ^{99m}Tc DTPA in a superficial vein distal to the suspected abnormality may also be used.

The standard for lower-extremity thrombus detection is the radiographic contrast venogram. Correlation between radionuclide venography and contrast venography has been reported to range from 77 to 96%. The limitations of the radionuclide venogram compared with contrast venography include nonvisualiza-

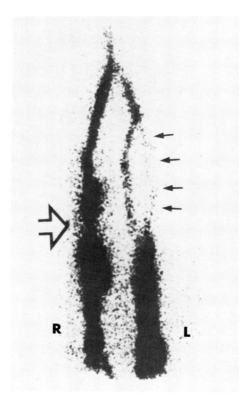

FIG. 5-5. Radionuclide venogram showing occlusion of the left femoral vein. A ghost of the left femoral vein can be seen (*small arrows*) with collateral flow through the saphenous system. The open arrow marks the popliteal area in the right lower extremity.

tion of the full extent of the thrombus as can be achieved with contrast venography, failure of radionuclide venography to detect nonocclusive and small thrombi as well as contrast venography, and false-positive results when collateral vessels are visualized but no active thrombosis is noted by contrast venography. The major disadvantage of the radiographic contrast venogram is that (1) it may be painful to the patient, particularly if there is any extravasation of the contrast, (2) <1% incidence of iatrogenic thrombosis induction, (3) the problem of potential reaction to contrast material, which carries a mortality rate of 1:40,000, and (4) potential renal toxicity.

Another test widely employed for the diagnosis of lower-extremity deep vein thrombosis is the ^{125}I fibrinogen uptake test. This test measures active deposition of fibrinogen. Since the radionuclide venogram discussed above does not distinguish old from new thrombi, the ^{125}I fibrinogen uptake may be a useful supplement in determining the age of an imaged clot.

Human fibrinogen labeled with ^{125}I is injected intravenously, and counts are obtained and recorded over multiple positions on both calves and thighs with a portable, hand-held scintillation detector. The lower-extremity counts are expressed as a percentage of the counts over the precordium. Focal increases of >20% compared with adjacent sites, with activity in the opposite leg, or with the same site at earlier times are interpreted as positive findings.

The fibrinogen uptake test is most sensitive for the detection of actively forming venous thrombosis, particularly in the calf. The test depends on incorporation of labeled fibrinogen into clots. This test has been most widely used prospectively in hospital patients at high risk for the development of deep vein thrombosis, such as elderly patients undergoing major abdominal operations. The test is less useful for the retrospective diagnosis of established deep vein thrombosis and in patients with suspected deep vein thrombosis in proximal femoral or iliac veins, the clot sites most commonly associated with pulmonary embolic disease.

Negative results do not exclude deep thrombophlebitis, and

contrast venography may still be required. False-positive results can occur with superficial thrombophlebitis, cellulitis, tissue injury, varicosities, and inflamed knee joints, all of which are accompanied by deposition of fibrinogen.

Another approach to detecting venous occlusive disease that does not require the often difficult cannulation of pedal veins is blood-pool imaging (Fig. 5-6) of the pelvis and lower extremities.

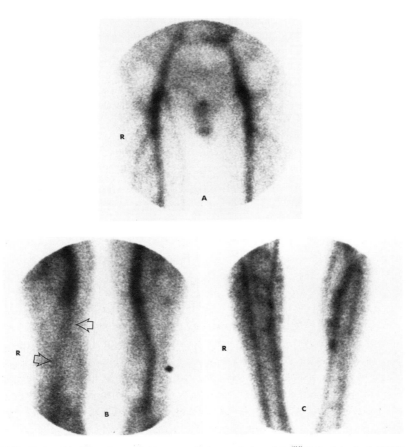

FIG. 5-6. (A) Blood-pool image of the pelvis with ^{99m}Tc-labeled RBC shows symmetric iliac vessels. (B) Blood-pool image of the thighs shows marked thinning of the right femoral–popliteal system in the adductor canal (*arrows*), indicating occlusive disease in this region. (C) Blood-pool image of the calves shows symmetric appearance of large vessels.

The patient's red cells are tagged with ^{99m}Tc pertechnetate, as outlined in Chapter 4, under gated cardiac blood-pool imaging. Access to any vein will suffice; the antecubital veins are used in most cases. Using the scintillation camera, stationary high-resolution images of the pelvic and lower extremity blood pool are obtained. Because the veins contain the largest volume of blood, they are the most prominently visualized vascular channels. Thrombosis is evident as an area of asymmetric decrease in vascular channel activity that may be accompanied by bridging superficial collateral channels. The technique does not distinguish between active or old occlusive venous disease; also, nonocclusive thrombosis may escape detection. Figure 5-6 shows a patient with occlusive changes in the right femoral vein.

A new agent being evaluated for imaging of venous thrombi, pulmonary emboli, arterial atherosclerotic lesions, and ventricular thrombi is ^{111}In platelets. Results of animal and human studies are thus far variable. Radiolabeled monoclonal antibodies directed against fibrin and fibrin products are also being investigated as potential agents for imaging thrombi and thromboemboli in patients.

SELECTED READINGS

Pulmonary Emboli

Alderson PO, Biello DR, Sachariah KG, Siegel BA. Scintigraphic detection of pulmonary embolism in patients with obstructive pulmonary disease. *Radiology* 1981; 138:661–666

Alderson PO, Doppman JL, Diamond SS, Mendenhall KG. Ventilation-perfusion imaging and selective pulmonary angiography in dogs with experimental pulmonary embolism. *J Nucl Med* 1978; 19:164–171

Alderson PO, Line BR. Scintigraphic evaluation of regional pulmonary ventilation. *Semin Nucl Med* 1980; 10:218–242

Alderson PO, Martin EC. Pulmonary embolism: Diagnosis with multiple imaging modalities. *Radiology* 1987; 164:297–312

Biello DR. Radiological (scintigraphic) evaluation of patients with suspected pulmonary thromboembolism. *JAMA* 1987; 257:3257–3259

Biello DR, Mattar AG, Osei-Wusu A, et al. Interpretation of indeterminate lung scintigrams. *Radiology* 1979; 133:189–194

Dalen JE, Albert JS. Natural history of pulmonary embolism. *Prog Cardiovasc Dis* 1975; 17(4):259–270

Hull RD, Hirsh J, Carter CJ, et al. Pulmonary angiography, ventilation lung scanning, and venography for clinically suspected pulmonary embolism with abnormal perfusion lung scan. *Ann Intern Med* 1983; 98:891–899

McNeil BJ. A diagnostic strategy using ventilation-perfusion studies in adults suspect for pulmonary embolism. *J Nucl Med* 1976; 17:613–616

McNeil BJ. Ventilation-perfusion studies and the diagnosis of pulmonary embolism. *J Nucl Med* 1980; 21:319–323

Moser KM, Harsanyi P, Ruise-Garriga G, et al. Assessment of pulmonary photoscanning and angiography in experimental pulmonary embolism. *Circulation* 1969; 39:663–673

Neumann RD, Sostman HD, Gottschalk A. Current status of ventilation-perfusion imaging. *Semin Nucl Med* 1980; 10:198–217

Thrombus Detection

DeNardo SJ. Role of nuclear medicine in the detection of venous thrombosis. In: Freeman LM, Weissmann HS, eds. *Nuclear medicine annual 1980.* New York: Raven Press; 1980:341–365

Games AS, Webber MM, Buffkin D. Contrast venography vs. radionuclide venography: A study of discrepancies and their possible significance. *Radiology* 1982; 142:719–728

Kakkar VV. Fibrinogen uptake test for detection of deep vein thrombosis—A review of current practice. *Semin Nucl Med* 1977; 7:229–244

Lisbona R. Radionuclide blood-pool imaging in the diagnosis of deep-vein thrombosis of the leg. In: Freeman LM, Weissmann HS, eds. *Nuclear medicine annual 1986.* New York: Raven Press; 1986:161–193

Moser KM, Brach BB, Dolan GF. Clinically suspected deep venous thrombosis of the lower extremities. A comparison of venography, impedance plethysmography and radiolabeled fibrinogen. *JAMA* 1977; 237:2195–2198

6

Liver and Gastrointestinal Tract

LIVER–SPLEEN IMAGING

Nuclear medicine techniques are more concerned with gastrointestinal (GI) function than with merely defining anatomy. Radionuclide liver–spleen scans are performed after intravenous administration of ^{99m}Tc labeled to a sulfur colloid that is trapped by the reticuloendothelial cells, most of which are located in the liver, spleen, and bone marrow. The radiocolloid liver scan provides an image of the functional behavior of reticuloendothelial cells that depends on cell numbers, distribution, integrity, and blood supply (Fig. 6-1).

Normally the bone narrow is not imaged on liver–spleen scans because of insufficient activity localization. However, in the presence of portal hypertension or liver disease, blood may be shunted from the portal to the systemic circulations, resulting in increased ^{99m}Tc colloid flowing to bone marrow and increased uptake sufficient for marrow visualization on routine images. In hepatocellular disease, changes in hepatic and splenic size and shape are also seen on the scan (Fig. 6-2).

Radionuclide liver scans are sensitive in detecting liver metastases and primary liver tumors imaged as regions of poor or absent radiocolloid (Fig. 6-3). In addition, liver scintigraphy is useful in localizing focal hepatic defects caused by abscesses, cysts, and trauma, as well as in confirming the absence of focal disease in patients found to have enlarged livers on physical

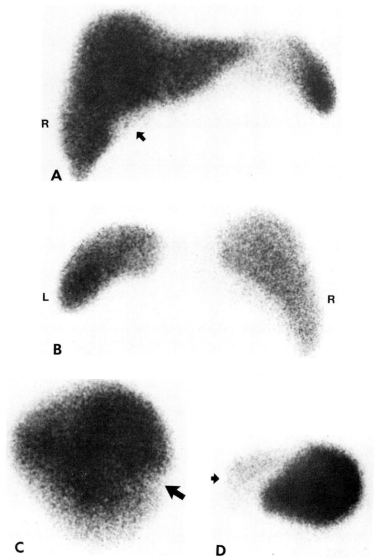

FIG. 6-1. Normal liver. (**A**) Anterior view shows prominent gallbladder fossa adjacent to portal area (*arrow*). (**B**) Posterior view shows uptake in liver on the right (*R*) and spleen on the left (*L*). (**C**) Right lateral view shows normal notch (*arrow*) along anterior hepatic surface. (**D**) Left lateral view shows prominent splenic activity posteriorly and a small bit of the left lobe of the liver anteriorly (*arrow*).

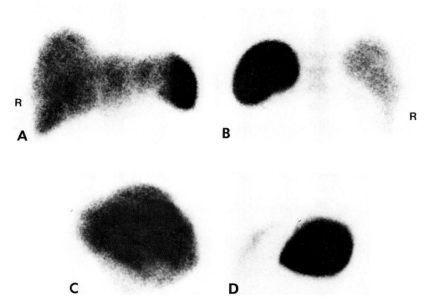

FIG. 6-2. Diffuse hepatocellular disease. (**A**) Anterior view shows a large liver with uneven uptake and relatively increased splenic uptake. (**B**) Posterior view shows increased uptake in a large spleen, poor hepatic uptake, and increased uptake in the vertebral marrow. (**C**) Right lateral view shows nonuniform hepatic uptake. (**D**) Left lateral view shows splenomegaly reflecting increased portal pressure secondary to longstanding hepatocellular disease.

examination. Thus, a focal defect on the liver scan is a nonspecific finding.

Whether a lesion is imaged on the liver–spleen scan depends mainly on the lesion size and shape, the depth of the lesion in tissue, and the inherent resolution limitations of the scintillation camera-collimator-film display imaging system. A 2.5-cm diameter lesion will probably be seen, even if it is deep within the liver. A 1.0-cm lesion might possibly be seen if it is near the liver surface and close to the camera, but would not be seen if it is buried deep within liver tissue. The chances of identifying a lesion deep within the liver are probably increased with SPECT imaging systems.

Reported sensitivity for detecting focal hepatic abnormali-

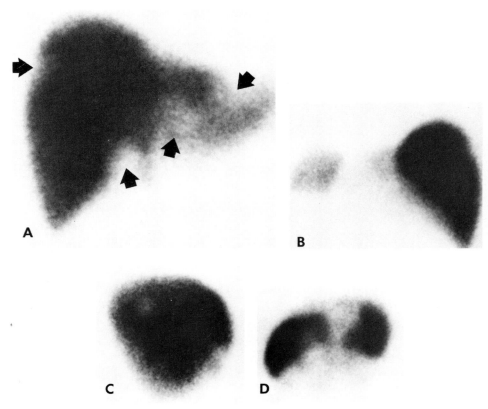

FIG. 6-3. Liver scan with multiple focal defects caused by metastases from esophageal carcinoma. (**A**) Anterior view shows multiple defects (*arrows*). (**B**) Posterior view shows only minimal indentations along lateral margin. (**C**) Right lateral view shows focal defect high in the superior–posterior aspect of the right lobe. (**D**) Left lateral view shows a defect in the posterior aspect of the left lobe.

ties by scintigraphy range from 50 to 95% and specificity from 46 to 97%. Likewise, comparisons between radiographic computed tomography (CT), ultrasound, and scintigraphy report wildly varying results. This variation partly reflects differences in populations selected for study, differing criteria for interpretation, variability in equipment for all modalities, variability in experimental designs, and bias.

Computed tomography has the capacity to define abnormalities in anatomically adjacent structures that may be pertinent to clinical management of the patient. Ultrasound images depend on tissue impedance differences and often characterize the nature of the detected lesion, particularly as cystic or solid.

Evaluation of computed tomographs may be hampered by individual patient characteristics, such as lack of fat to define tissue planes, inability to hold still or to lie flat, inability to hold one's breath, and allergy to radiographic contrast media or renal failure contraindicating its use. Likewise, for sonography, such factors as bowel gas, marked obesity, and dressings, wounds, or appliances that interfere with transducer-to-skin coupling may hamper examination.

A combination of imaging modalities may be the optimum approach to identifying and characterizing liver lesions. For example, after a lesion has been identified on CT, delayed ^{99m}Tc RBC imaging can specifically characterize a hemangioma because of delayed pooling of activity. The choice of imaging modalities used will vary from one institution to another, often depending on availability of equipment and expertise as well as cost.

ESOPHAGUS, STOMACH, AND DUODENUM

Scintigraphic Esophageal Transit Studies

Esophageal symptoms range from nonspecific complaints to frank pain or obstruction, or both, related to esophageal erosions or cancer. Many disorders of the esophagus are associated with abnormalities in esophageal transit.

Until recently, a sensitive noninvasive test to evaluate esophageal transit was not available. Radionuclide methods have now been developed that employ an oral tracer dose of ^{99m}Tc sulfur colloid, detected using a scintillation camera on-line to a digital computer. This technique both objectively and physiologically measures the transit time of a radioactive bolus through the esophagus.

The scintigraphic techniques have been compared with radiographic methods, manometric methods, and endoscopy and are more sensitive for detecting and quantitating abnormalities of esophageal transit. Clinically, scintigraphy is useful in patients with achalasia, scleroderma, diffuse esophageal spasm, and nonspecific motor disorders of the esophagus, and in patients with reflux esophagitis. These techniques are employed for diagnosis and follow-up in patients treated either medically or surgically.

Gastroesophageal Reflux

Patients with gastroesophageal reflux (and some without) complain of heartburn resulting from the retrograde movement of gastric and duodenal contents across the gastroesophageal junction, causing inflammation of the distal esophageal mucosa. The clinical picture is sometimes atypical, and the response to treatment may not be uniformly satisfactory.

Although upper GI contrast studies and endoscopy are first used to exclude other processes, such as cancer or peptic ulcer disease, scintigraphy is the most sensitive imaging technique in detecting gastroesophageal reflux as the cause of symptoms. The method employs ^{99m}Tc sulfur colloid administered orally and imaged using a scintillation camera on-line to a digital computer. The patient is stressed during the study by being placed in a supine position, being given acidified fluid with the tracer dose, and applying an inflatable abdominal binder to induce an artificial Valsalva-like maneuver.

Gastroesophageal scintigraphy is more sensitive than radiographic, endoscopic, or manometric techniques and is the first quantitative test of gastroesophageal reflux. The technique measures the percentage of activity initially present in the stomach that regurgitates into the esophagus at varying pressures.

Pulmonary Aspiration Studies

In order to document occult pulmonary aspiration of gastric contents, an insoluble tracer such as ^{99m}Tc sulfur colloid may be instilled in the stomach at bedtime, and imaging of the pulmonary area is performed the following morning. Clumps of activity in the lung-field indicate aspiration.

Gastric Emptying

Most studies of gastric emptying are deficient in that they are not quantitative or are relatively invasive (e.g., intubation), hence uncomfortable for the patient. By contrast, radionuclide methods permit administration of physiologic meals of defined calorie content, weight, and volume, with sequential quantitative imaging. The study measures the half-time disappearance of a labeled liquid or solid meal from the stomach. Deviation from established normal ranges permits identification and quantitation of abnormal gastric emptying and gastroparesis in patients with diabetes or in those who have undergone surgical or pharmacologic therapy. In addition to diagnosis, this test is used as an objective tool to monitor response to therapy. These physiologic studies provide increased sensitivity of gastric emptying analysis.

Bile Reflux Scintigraphy

Using a radionuclidic agent concentrated in the gallbladder, such as one of the iminodiacetic acid (IDA) compounds (see Chapter 7), reflux of bile from the small bowel into the stomach and esophagus can be imaged. After intravenous administration of the hepatobiliary agent and visualization of the gallbladder, the patient's endogenous cholecystokinin (CCK) is stimulated by means of a fatty meal or exogenous CCK to stimulate emptying of the gallbladder. Sequential imaging of the gallbladder and stomach is then performed in an effort to identify reflux of bile from the small bowel into the stomach. This physiologic method of identifying bile reflux is also quantifiable using a scintillation camera interfaced to a computer. The degree of bile reflux imaged by this technique correlates with the severity of symptoms in patients after surgery for peptic ulcer disease.

Ectopic Gastric Mucosa

In Barrett's esophagus, columnar epithelium resembling that in the stomach is found in the distal portion of the esophagus. Technetium-99m pertechnetate is concentrated in the mucus-producing glands of the stomach and can therefore be used to identify ectopic gastric mucosa found in the esophagus or elsewhere. This approach is used less often now that endoscopy is routinely employed, but may be useful in specific clinical situations. Similarly, ectopic gastric mucosa in enterogenous thoracic cysts and Meckel's diverticula may be readily detected by the uptake of ^{99m}Tc pertechnetate.

Meckel's Diverticulum

Meckel's diverticulum is a common anomaly present in 2–3% of the population. Although most persons who have this anomaly remain asymptomatic throughout life, they can present with bleeding, diverticulitis, intestinal obstruction due to intussusception, and volvulus. Approximately 50% of complications occur in children less than 2 yr old. Adults more often present with diverticulitis or obstruction, while children are more likely to present with bleeding.

This anomaly is found in the ileum, usually within 45 cm (18 in.) of the ileocecal valve. Pathologically, the wall of the diverticulum may contain aberrant tissue identical to gastric mucosa. Therefore, it can be identified on radionuclide images following intravenous injection of ^{99m}Tc pertechnetate, which is rapidly and actively secreted by gastric mucosa.

Autoradiographic studies indicate that pertechnetate is concentrated and secreted by the epithelial cells, rather than the parietal cells of the stomach. If the patient presents with bleeding, the alternative radionuclide imaging approach using ^{99m}Tc sulfur colloid or ^{99m}Tc-labeled red blood cells (RBCs) to identify a site of GI bleeding may be used, and then followed by a ^{99m}Tc pertechnetate Meckel's scan (see section below on Acute Gastrointestinal Hemorrhage). Imaging with ^{99m}Tc pertechnetate is reported to have an overall accuracy of 85–95% in detecting Meckel's diverticulum.

Gastrointestinal Function Tests

Nonimaging in vitro tests of gastrointestinal function include the Schilling test (see Chapter 14) for pernicious anemia, stool studies for fat malabsorption and slow GI blood loss, and breath tests for fat malabsorption and bacterial overgrowth in the small bowel.

ACUTE GASTROINTESTINAL HEMORRHAGE

Radionuclide techniques for detecting GI bleeding sites have been validated experimentally and used clinically. The alternative imaging procedure to localize the site of GI bleeding is radiographic angiography. In addition to its superior sensitivity for identifying active GI bleeding, the radionuclide study may be a valuable guide for selective abdominal arteriography. Either intravenously administered ^{99m}Tc sulfur colloid or ^{99m}Tc-labeled RBCs are used. The colloid is cleared rapidly mainly by the liver and spleen, so that the fraction of the injected activity that extravasates at the active GI bleeding site may be seen as a "hot" focus. Because there is rapid clearance of the agent from the vascular system by the liver and spleen, the contrast of bleeding site to surrounding tissue is high if the bleeding site is not in the field of the liver or spleen. But bleeding must occur during the few minutes after injection if it is to be detected, while the blood level of the radiocolloid is high. Therefore, intermittent bleeding may be missed. Published reports indicate that bleeding sites were detectable at bleeding rates as low as 0.1 ml/min in animal studies in which the rate of bleeding was controlled. Clinically, this approach is useful in active lower GI tract bleeding in both diagnostic localization and for following the efficacy of therapy.

Although the ^{99m}Tc sulfur colloid approach has the advantage of a clean lower abdominal background for imaging a focal bleeding site, the ^{99m}Tc RBC approach offers the opportunity to detect intermittent bleeding over a 24-hr period and to detect upper GI bleeding in the region of the liver and spleen, which cannot be visualized by the colloid technique. Both the ^{99m}Tc-labeled RBCs and ^{99m}Tc sulfur colloid appear to be more sensitive than angiography, which reportedly detects bleeding rates of 0.5 ml/min (as compared with 0.1 ml/min).

Using the labeled RBC technique, serial imaging over a 24-hr period can be performed, as the labeled material remains in the circulating blood. As the activity continues to leak from the blood at the bleeding site, enough accumulates to permit detection. It must be noted that normal bowel peristalsis may displace the activity distally from the original site of deposition, which can result in misjudgment of the actual bleeding site. To prevent this from occurring it is advisable to continue imaging at frequent intervals (every 2–3 hr) for the duration of the study.

A pitfall of this technique is gastric or colonic concentration of free ^{99m}Tc pertechnetate that has broken off from labeled cells and is concentrated in gastric secretions. From the stomach, the pertechnetate moves distally in the gut. Without the benefit of frequent serial images, this activity can be mistaken for an active bleeding site.

SELECTED READINGS

General Gastrointestinal

Chadudhuri TK. Gastrointestinal imaging with radionuclides. In: Freeman LM, Weissmann HS, eds. *Nuclear medicine annual 1983*. New York: Raven Press; 1983:199–230

Liver-Spleen Imaging

Drum DE. Current status of radiocolloid hepatic scintiphotography for space-occupying disease. *Semin Nucl Med* 1982; 12:64–74

Patton DD. Current status of liver scintigraphy for space-occupying disease. In: Freeman LM, Weissmann HS, eds. *Nuclear medicine annual 1982*. New York: Raven Press; 1982:35–80

Waxman AD. Scintigraphic evaluation of diffuse hepatic disease. *Semin Nucl Med* 1982; 12:75–88

Esophageal Transit and Gastrointestinal Reflux

Malmud LS, Fisher RS. Radionuclide studies of esophageal transit and gastroesophageal reflux. *Semin Nucl Med* 1982; 12:104–125

Gastric Emptying

Christian PE, Moore JG, Soreson JA, et al. Effects of meal size and correction technique on gastric emptying time: Studies with two tracers and opposed detectors. *J Nucl Med* 1980; 21:883–885

Pulmonary Aspiration

Boonyaprapa S, Alderson PO, Garfinkel D, et al. Detection of pulmonary aspiration in infants and children with respiratory disease. *J Nucl Med* 1980; 21:214–218

Bile Reflux Scintigraphy

Rosenthall L, Shaffer EA, Lisbona R, et al. Diagnosis of hepatobiliary disease by Tc-99m HIDA cholescintigraphy. *Radiology* 1978; 126:467–474

Ectopic Gastric Mucosa

Berquest TH, Nolan NG, Stephens DH, et al. Radioisotope scintigraphy in diagnosis of Barrett's esophagus. *Am J Roentgenol Rad Ther Nucl Med* 1975; 123:401–411

Sfakianakis GN, Conway JJ. Detection of ectopic gastric mucosa in Meckel's diverticulum and in other aberrations by scintigraphy. II. Indications and methods—A 10-year experience. *J Nucl Med* 1981; 22:732–1981

Meckel's Diverticulum

Conway JJ. Radionuclide diagnosis of Meckel's diverticulum. *Gastrointest Radiol* 1980; 5:209–213

Kilpatrick ZM. Scanning in diagnosis of Meckel's diverticulum. *Hosp Pract* 1974; 9:131–139

Taylor AT, Alazraki N, Henry JE. Intestinal concentration of ^{99m}Tc-pertechnetate into isolated loops of rat bowel. *J Nucl Med* 1976; 17:470–472

Gastrointestinal Function Tests

Reba RC, Salkeled J. In-vitro studies of malabsorption and other GI disorders. *Semin Nucl Med* 1982; 12:147–155

Acute Gastrointestinal Hemorrhage

Alavi A. Detection of gastrointestinal bleeding with ^{99m}Tc sulfur colloid. *Semin Nucl Med* 1982; 17:126–138

Wenzelbergg GG, McKusick KA, Froelich JW, et al. Detection of gastrointestinal bleeding with ^{99m}Tc-labeled red blood cells. *Semin Nucl Med* 1982; 12:139–146

7
Biliary Tract

The introduction of the ^{99m}Tc-labeled iminodiacetic acid (IDA) compounds (^{99m}Tc IDA) permits a noninvasive means of analyzing hepatobiliary disorders. These agents are extracted from the blood by the hepatocytes and are concentrated in bile. The ^{99m}Tc IDA study provides an image of hepatocyte function and outlines the pathway of bile flow. Biliary tree visualization may be obtained even in some rare cases with bilirubin levels as high as 30 mg%. At many medical centers ^{99m}Tc IDA cholescintigraphy is the procedure of choice for diagnosing the cystic duct obstruction that almost invariably accompanies acute cholecystitis. It sensitively detects significant common duct obstruction, particularly in the acute phase, as well as biliary leaks. The images can define the altered anatomy and physiology that result after cholecystectomy and surgical diversionary shunts.

The technique involves obtaining serial images of the abdomen, including the right upper quadrant after intravenous injection of ^{99m}Tc IDA in patients prepared by fasting at least 4 hr. Normally the liver, common bile duct, gallbladder, duodenum, and jejunum are visualized on the images obtained within 60 min (Fig. 7-1).

CHOLECYSTITIS

Acute

The key diagnostic question in suspected acute cholecystitis is patency versus obstruction of the cystic duct. The sensitivity of

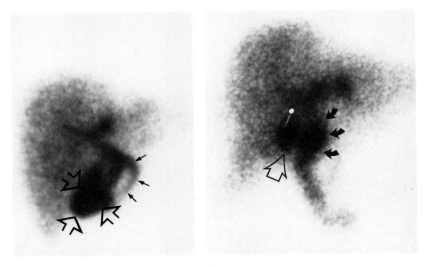

A   **B**

FIG. 7-1. Normal hepatobiliary study. (**A**) 10 min after i.v. injection the liver has extracted the major portion of the ^{99m}Tc IDA agent from the blood. Activity delineates the hepatic ducts, common duct (*small arrows*) to the duodenum, and gallbladder (*open arrow*) nestled adjacent to the duodenum. (**B**) This 30-min image shows activity in the gall bladder (*open arrow*), common duct (*curved arrows*) as well as in the small bowel and in the left side of the abdomen.

^{99m}Tc IDA cholescintigraphy in making this determination exceeds 95%, and the specificity approaches 99%, leading to an overall accuracy of >97% in the acute situation. Accuracy falls in certain clinical situations, such as alcoholic liver disease and hyperalimentation. While some small series have reported that pancreatitis can be a cause of nonvisualization of the gallbladder, the preponderance of data suggests that the test is accurate in cases of pancreatitis.

Judicious use of cholecystokinin prior to study of patients who have been fasting for prolonged periods may increase the accuracy of the ^{99m}Tc IDA study. Similarly, intravenous (i.v.) administration of a low dose of morphine after visualization of the common duct and duodenum may enhance gallbladder filling by constricting the sphincter of Oddi and increase accuracy.

Safety and reliability of ^{99m}Tc IDA imaging exceeds that of i.v. contrast cholangiography, which has a false-positive rate of 12–22%, cannot visualize a patent biliary tree when the serum bilirubin begins to rise above 2–4 mg%, and has a significant morbidity and mortality.

Ultrasound provides anatomic information simply, safely, and rapidly. However, as a purely morphologic imaging modality, it too has limitations for the diagnosis of acute cholecystitis. Ultrasound is extremely sensitive in detecting cholelithiasis but, since estimates suggest that 20 million Americans have gallstones, finding them cannot automatically be equated with acute cholecystitis. Gallstones may be incidental findings in patients with other causes of acute upper abdominal pain, fever, and leukocytosis. The ultrasonic demonstration of gallbladder wall thickening caused by edema, a pericholecystic collection, or a gallstone in the cystic duct (which typically is difficult to visualize sonographically) can provide a specific diagnosis of acute cholecystitis. However, these findings are much less consistently observed in patients with acute cholecystitis than is gallbladder nonvisualization by scintigraphy (Fig. 7-2).

Cholescintigraphy also has a significant advantage with regard to the diagnosis of acute acalculous cholecystitis. Depending on the expertise and bias of a particular institution, cholescintigraphy or ultrasound is done first in the workup of patients with suspected acute cholecystitis.

Chronic

The role of ^{99m}Tc IDA imaging in diagnosing chronic cholecystitis is limited for three reasons: First, it cannot provide a direct answer to the key question: Are gallstones present?—the finding most commonly associated with chronic cholecystitis. Ultrasound and oral cholecystography, on the other hand, answer this question accurately. Second, patients with chronic cholecystitis usually have a patent biliary tree; therefore, a normal cholescintigram

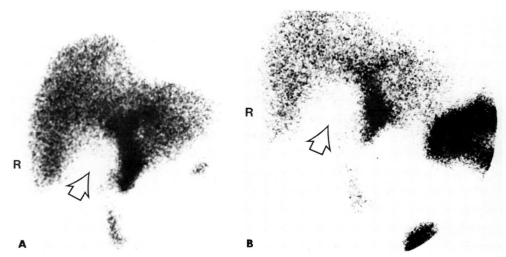

FIG. 7-2. Acute cholecystitis with nonvisualization of the gallbladder on the ^{99m}Tc IDA study. (**A**) This 10-min anterior image shows the hepatic ducts and a large empty space (*arrow*) in the gallbladder fossa. The common duct has already begun emptying into the duodenum. (**B**) After 1 hr has elapsed, a magnified view shows the liver has emptied most of its activity into the small bowel, although the hepatic ducts can still be seen. The gallbladder still is not filled (*arrow*), indicating cystic duct obstruction that is almost invariably associated with acute cholecystitis.

does not exclude chronic cholecystitis. Third, a wide spectrum of cholescintigraphic patterns occurs, depending on the presence of either partial or complete functional cystic or common duct obstruction by stones or sludge, or both.

Although delayed gallbladder visualization with ^{99m}Tc IDA is highly suggestive, it is not pathognomonic of chronic cholecystitis. The cholescintigram can be helpful in evaluating the patient with known cholelithiasis presenting with acute abdominal pain and occasionally in the patient in whom other studies have shown no abnormal findings (false-negative) but for whom the clinical findings strongly suggest chronic cholecystitis.

BILIARY LEAKAGE

Technetium-99m IDA provides a sensitive means of identifying, localizing, and permitting serial evaluation of biliary leaks. After surgery, the preferential route of bile flow can be traced, whether through a surgical anastomosis or into an abnormal collection, without introduction of nonphysiologic artifacts from pressure injection through catheters or risk of infection and other complications.

CHOLESTASIS

Ultrasound or x-ray computed tomography (CT) accurately detect biliary ductal dilatation and frequently determine the level and cause of obstruction. In specific instances, biliary scintigraphy may be useful in cases of acute common bile duct obstruction when functional stasis is detectable before dilatation, and occasionally, even before liver function tests become abnormal. It is also useful in cases of localized intrahepatic ductal obstruction. Technetium-99m IDA imaging can be used to distinguish nonobstructive from obstructive jaundice, but CT and ultrasound provide better accuracy.

POSTOPERATIVE EVALUATION

Whereas ultrasound gives accurate anatomic information, ^{99m}Tc IDA hepatobiliary imaging provides evaluation of functional patency as well as the capability for detecting cystic duct remnants and postoperative bile leaks. The functional information thus obtained complements sonography. It also routinely visualizes a patent surgical anastomosis at any level, such as hepaticoduodenostomy, cholecystojejunostomy, or choledochojejunostomy, even though the sphincter of Oddi has been bypassed. In this situation, x-ray contrast media may fail to trace the pathway of bile flow. The location and size of an anastomotic bile leak can therefore be physiologically imaged on the nuclear scan, while other approaches, including the T-tube study, percutaneous cholangiography, and the upper gastrointestinal series using barium, are nonphysiologic. The normal reflux of air into the biliary ducts in these patients interferes with sonographic evaluation, but not with cholescintigraphy.

TRAUMA

Cholescintigraphy is well suited for the evaluation of biliary fistulas or leakage in patients with blunt abdominal injuries, as this technique does not require the presence of a tract communicating with the skin surface. Serial studies in cases of biliary leakage provide accurate evaluation of spontaneous resolution or response to therapy.

SELECTED READINGS

General

Weissmann HS. Cholescintigraphy. In: Berk RN, Ferrucci JT, Jr, and Leopold G, eds. *Radiology of the gallbladder and bile ducts: Diagnosis and intervention.* Philadelphia: WB Saunders; 1983:261–313

Acute Cholecystitis

Freeman LM, Weissmann HS, Rosenblatt R, Freitas JE. Correspondence regarding ultrasound versus radionuclide imaging in the evaluation of patients with acute right upper quadrant pain. *Radiology* 1982; 143:280–282

Freitas JE, Gulati RM. Rapid evaluation of acute abdominal pain by hepatobiliary scanning. *JAMA* 1980; 244:1585–1587

Weissmann HS, Badia J, Sugarman LA, et al. Spectrum of 99m-Tc-IDA cholescintigraphic patterns in acute cholecystitis. *Radiology* 1981; 138:167–175

Biliary Leakage

Christensen PB, Oester-Jorgensen E, Schoubye J, et al. Scintigraphy with 99m-Tc-(2,6-diethyl-acetanilide)-iminodiacetic acid as a diagnostic test in traumatic lesions of the liver and biliary tract. *Gastrointest Radiol* 1981; 6:43–46

Weissmann HS, Byun KJC, Freeman LM. Role of Tc-99m IDA scintigraphy in the evaluation of hepatobiliary trauma. *Semin Nucl Med* 1983; 13:199–222

Cholestasis

Scharschmidt BF, Goldberg HI, Schmid R. Current concepts in diagnosis: Approach to the patient with cholestatic jaundice. *N Engl J Med* 1983; 308:1515–1519

Weissmann HS, Rosenblatt R, Sugarman LA, et al. The role of nuclear imaging in evaluating the patient with cholestasis. *Semin Ultrasound* 1980; 1:134–142

Postoperative Evaluation

Rosenthall L, Fonseca C, Arzoumanian A, et al. 99m-Tc-IDA hepatobiliary imaging following upper abdominal surgery. *Radiology* 1979; 130:735–739

Weissmann HS, Gliedman ML, Wilk PJ, et al. Evaluation of the postoperative patient with 99m-Tc-IDA cholescintigraphy. *Semin Nucl Med* 1982; 12:27–52

8
Genitourinary Tract

The availability of ^{131}I hippurate and other ^{99m}Tc compounds provides a rapid, completely safe means of evaluating suspected renal and testicular disorders. Ideally, before any diagnostic test is obtained, it is important to have a specific clinical question in mind. Once the question is formulated, it is important to pick the diagnostic test(s) that best provide the answer.

The information that can be obtained by renal scintigraphy may be summarized as follows:

1. Determine relative renal function in patients with asymmetric renal disease.
2. Distinguish nonobstructed dilatation of the renal pelvis from dilation caused by mechanical obstruction.
3. Evaluate the vascular supply to the kidneys in patients with renal trauma, dissecting aneurysm, and other disorders.
4. Detect ureteral reflux in pediatric patients or patients with neurogenic bladder.
5. Distinguish a renal column of Bertin from a true mass.
6. Determine renal morphology and function in patients allergic to x-ray contrast media.
7. Identify patients with possible renovascular hypertension.
8. Evaluate the kidneys of patients with renal transplant for the complications of infarction, leakage, obstruction, acute tubular necrosis, and rejection.

EVALUATION OF RENAL FUNCTION

The most common measurement of renal function is the creatinine clearance. Often this determination is sufficient, but the creatinine clearance is a global index and provides no information regarding regional or relative function of the two kidneys. Measurement of individual kidney function can provide important diagnostic and prognostic information in patients with known or suspected renal disease. It can aid the urologist before renal surgery by providing quantitative relative function data for any region of either kidney. This may be particularly important when the surgical question is one of nephrectomy versus a reconstructive procedure.

The classic method for quantitating individual renal function requires cystoscopy and ureteral catheterization. This invasive technique is uncomfortable, potentially risky to the patient, expensive, and it may well be inaccurate because of contamination of urine with blood or seepage of urine around the catheter. Radiographic intravenous contrast media pyelography or urography defines renal anatomy rather than function, and this study may occasionally cause deterioration of renal function, particularly in the elderly patient with preexisting renal disease. Rarely, a potentially lethal contrast reaction may occur.

Radionuclide renal imaging is an accurate technique for evaluating individual renal function. It should be remembered, however, that the term "renal function scanning" does not refer to the existence of a single parameter of global function that can be measured by a scan and accurately partitioned between the two kidneys. Such a concept is an oversimplification. There are a number of parameters of renal function, all of which reflect the kidney's role in the formation of urine.

Radiopharmaceuticals for Renal Function Studies

A qualitative assessment of renal perfusion can be made after a bolus injection of any ^{99m}Tc complex. Iodine-I-131 hippuran

(OIH) is structurally similar to p-aminohippurate (PAH) and is cleared primarily by the renal tubules. Hippuran excretion measures the effective renal plasma flow (ERPF). Iodine-I-123-hippuran is now commercially available and is handled by the kidney the same as ^{131}I hippuran. Because of its lower photon energy (159 keV) and absence of β-emission, ^{123}I provides better renal images with less radiation to the patient but is considerably more expensive than ^{131}I hippuran. Technetium-99m mercaptoacetyltriglycine (MAG$_3$) is a new technetium radiopharmaceutical under development that should be commercially available within 1–2 yrs. Technetium-99m MAG$_3$ is handled by the kidney similarly to OIH.

Technetium-99m DTPA (diethylenetriamine pentaacetic acid) is cleared by the glomerulus in the same manner as inulin and can be used to measure the glomerular filtration rate (GFR). In a well-hydrated patient, GFR can be measured using ^{99m}Tc DTPA or ^{125}I iothalamate infusion or subcutaneous injection in order to attain a constant plasma level during the time that urine is collected for counting. GFR can also be determined from multiple blood samples following a bolus injection. In most nuclear medicine departments, GFR is estimated from a single timed blood sample or the radioactivity accumulated in the kidney 2–3 min postinjection. ERPF can be determined using similar techniques following ^{131}I OIH administration.

Technetium-99m DMSA (dimercaptosuccinic acid) binds to the renal tubules and provides an image of cortical anatomy; the relative distribution of DMSA between the two kidneys is a measure of relative renal blood flow and tubular function.

Technetium-99m glucoheptonate and ^{99m}Tc iron ascorbate DTPA are cleared by both glomerular filtration and tubular excretion. Because approximately 10% of the dose remains in the renal parenchyma, good cortical images can also be obtained.

In summary, several radiopharmaceuticals can be used to measure relative renal function. Measurements of total GFR and ERPF can also be obtained. In practice, it may be useful to discuss each case with the nuclear medicine physician in order to tailor the study to specific clinical requirements.

HYDRONEPHROSIS OR POSSIBLE OBSTRUCTION

Hydronephrosis, the dilatation of the renal pelvis and/or collecting system, is often caused by obstruction which may be detected using a variety of agents. Figure 8-1 shows a ^{99m}Tc glucoheptonate study in a patient with a left ureterovesical stone causing acute partial obstruction. Figure 8-2 shows a Hippuran® study, both

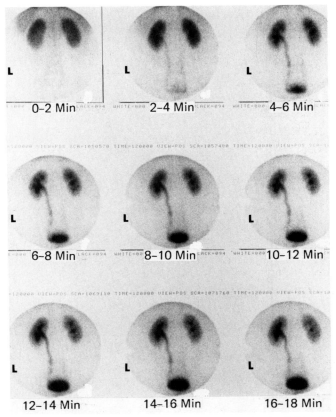

FIG. 8-1. Serial posterior images obtained every 2 min following injection of ^{99m}Tc glucoheptonate in a patient with partial obstruction of drainage from the left kidney due to a stone lodged at the left ureterovesical junction. Persistent activity can be seen in the left renal pelvis and ureter whereas the right side fills and empties normally.

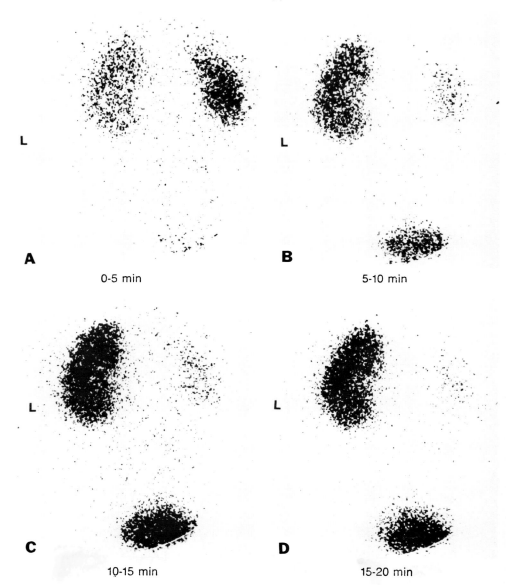

FIG. 8-2 (A–D) Serial posterior 5-min hippuran images in a patient with obstruction of the left ureter due to a stone show poor initial concentration by the left kidney and then retention when the normal right kidney has emptied. Bladder activity appears at the bottom of images **A–D**.

106

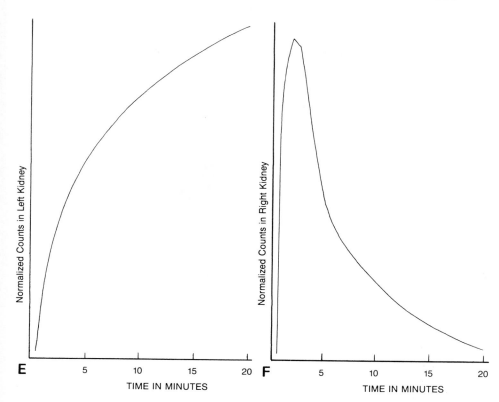

FIG. 8-2. (E-F) The renogram curves of ^{131}I hippuran activity in the kidneys on the ordinate and time on the abscissa show an ascending curve on the left, **E**, characteristic of obstruction, and a normal right curve, **F**.

images and renogram curves, in another patient with left-sided obstruction due to a stone lodged in the left ureterovesical junction. If obstruction persists, surgical intervention is usually indicated. The diuretic-augmented renogram is an excellent test for distinguishing nonobstructive versus obstructive dilatation of the renal pelvis. The test can also be useful to determine whether surgery has been successful in relieving a known obstruction and to evaluate recovery of function in the damaged kidney.

The study is commonly performed by injecting the patient

with 370–740 MBq (10–20 mCi) ^{99m}Tc DTPA. The radiopharmaceutical is cleared by GFR, permitting visualization of the pelvocalyceal system. If there is good renal uptake and the radiopharmaceutical clears the collecting system spontaneously in 20–30 min, no obstruction is present. If there is marked retention in the collecting system, the patient is given furosemide (usually 0.3 mg/kg for the adult), and imaging is continued. Prompt clearance of the radionuclide from the pelvis is the normal response. If the radionuclide activity in the pelvis increases, obstruction is present. The method is not valid, however, if the kidney under evaluation is severely damaged, because a poorly functioning kidney may not respond to furosemide with a significant diuresis.

URETERAL REFLUX

A large number of pediatric patients are seen because of repeated urinary tract infection and vesicoureteral reflux. Once a contrast study has been obtained to document reflux and define anatomy, the patient should be followed by radionuclide cystography, as the technique is quite accurate for detecting reflux, and the radiation dose to the patient and gonads is much less than with a contrast study.

The study is usually performed by instilling saline containing a ^{99m}Tc radiopharmaceutical into the bladder through a catheter. Imaging is performed continuously during filling of the bladder and subsequent voiding. By recording data on a computer, both reflux and the voiding volume can be quantitated.

RENAL PARENCHYMAL MASSES

Excellent anatomic images of the kidneys can be obtained using ^{99m}Tc DMSA or glucoheptonate in patients with allergies to contrast media or in those with a relative contraindication to contrast media administration. Most renal masses, whether cyst, neoplasm or abscess, fail to concentrate radiopharmaceuticals used for renal imaging. They appear as areas of decreased activity, indistinguishable from one another. A renal column of Bertin is composed of normal cortical tissue, but it can appear as a questionable mass on an intravenous urogram. The presence of normal cortical tissue can be confirmed by a renal scan with an agent such as ^{99m}Tc DMSA, which shows concentration of the radiopharmaceutical corresponding to the questionable area on the intravenous urogram.

RENOVASCULAR HYPERTENSION

Renal scans can be useful in evaluating the patient suspected of having renovascular hypertension and in predicting the effect of angioplasty on renal function. The efficacy of renal imaging as a screening method for renovascular hypertension is critically dependent on prevalence as well as technique and varying results have been reported in the literature. Renal scans following administration of the angiotensin-converting enzyme inhibitor, captopril, are reported to increase the sensitivity and specificity of the renal scan in detecting renovascular hypertension. Experimental studies in animals have shown that when renal artery blood flow is diminished to 50% of the normal baseline level, radionuclide imaging and renogram techniques detect the abnormality. However, more work is needed to establish clearly the role and limitations of this technique.

RENAL TRANSPLANTATION

Complications of renal transplantation include parenchymal failure attributable to acute tubular necrosis (ATN), rejection, mechanical failure caused by injury to the renal artery or vein, partial or complete ureteral obstruction, and extravasation, which can usually be detected by renal scanning. A normal post-transplant scan excludes these complications.

Serial scans during the first 1–3 weeks post-transplantation can be used to monitor recovery from post-transplantation ATN and may also detect early rejection 24–48 hr before biochemical abnormalities occur.

SCROTAL IMAGING
(TORSION VERSUS EPIDIDYMITIS)

Spermatic cord torsion is a medical emergency, and prompt surgical exploration is necessary to salvage the involved testis. The cause of acute unilateral testicular swelling and pain is usually torsion of the spermatic cord or acute epididymitis. Other possibilities include torsion of the testicular appendage, orchitis, strangulated hernia, or hemorrhage. The use of radionuclide scrotal imaging enables the surgeon to avoid unnecessary surgery in patients with acute epididymitis and to proceed to prompt surgical exploration in patients with probable torsion.

The study can be performed within 10–15 min. The patient is given a bolus injection of ^{99m}Tc pertechnetate, and a radionuclide angiogram of testicular perfusion is obtained. Additional images are obtained immediately after the perfusion study has been performed. An area of decreased vascularity corresponding to the involved testis indicates that torsion is likely. If the clinically involved testis is normally perfused or hypervascular, emergency surgery is unnecessary. Adequate examinations will detect more than 95% of patients with torsion; 80–85% of patients with nontorsion will be correctly identified and spared unnecessary surgery.

SELECTED READINGS

Renal Scanning

Ash JM, Antico VG, Gilday DL, Houle S. Special consideration in the pediatric use of radionuclides for kidney studies. *Semin Nucl Med* 1982; 12(4):345–369

Dubovsky EV, Russell CD. Quantitation of renal function with glomerular and tubular agents. *Semin Nucl Med* 1982; 12:308–329

Kirchner PT, Rosenthall L. Renal transplant evaluation. *Semin Nucl Med* 1982; 12(4):370–378

Koff SA, Thrall SH, Keyes JW Jr. Diuretic radionuclide urography: A noninvasive method for evaluating nephroureteral dilatation. *J Urol* 1979; 122:451–454

O'Reilly PH, Shields RA, Testa HJ (eds). *Nuclear medicine in urology and nephrology*, 2nd ed. London: Butterworths; 1986

Tauxe WN, Dubovsky EV, Kidd T Jr, et al. New formulae for the calculation of effective renal plasma flow. *Eur J Nucl Med* 1982; 7:51–54

Tauxe WN and Dubovsky E (eds). *Nuclear medicine in clinical urology and nephrology*. Norwalk, CT: Appleton & Lange; 1985

Taylor A Jr. Quantitation of renal function with static imaging agents. *Semin Nucl Med* 1977; 2:173–177

Taylor AT Jr. Quantitative renal function scanning: A historical and current status report on renal radiopharmaceuticals. In: Freeman LM, Weissmann HS, eds. *Nuclear medicine annual 1980*. New York: Raven Press; 1980:303–341

Ureteral Reflux

Conway JJ. Radionuclide cystography. In: Tauxe WN, Dubovsky EV, eds. *Nuclear medicine in clinical urology and nephrology*. Norwalk, CT: Appleton & Lange; 1985:305–320

Scrotal Imaging

Holder LE, Melloul M, Chen D. Current status of radionuclide scrotal imaging. *Semin Nucl Med* 1981; 11:232–249

Lutzker LG. The fine points of scrotal scintigraphy. *Semin Nucl Med* 1982; 12:387–393

Tanaka T, Mishkin F, Datta NS. Radionuclide imaging of the scrotal contents. In: Freeman LS, Weissmann HS, eds. *Nuclear medicine annual 1981*. New York: Raven Press; 1981:195–222

9

Skeletal System

PRINCIPLES OF RADIONUCLIDE BONE IMAGING

Radionuclide bone images display incorporation of a radiopharmaceutical into the skeletal structure, reflecting the histologic events of osteogenesis. By contrast, roentgenographic methods record the x-rays transmitted through bone, which depends on the mineral content of bone, chiefly calcium. The higher the bone mineral content, the greater the absorption of x-rays and the lower the transmission of x-rays.

Since the bone scan and bone radiograph reflect different properties of bone, it should not be surprising that the results of bone scans and radiographs diverge in varying disease states. The response of bone to any insult, trauma, ischemia, infection, or neoplasm is to repair itself by activating its cellular constituents, the osteoblast, osteoclast, and osteocyte, to accelerate the remodeling process. Bone formation and resorption occur simultaneously and the end result is not a function of the particular process that activates this cycle, but rather of the net balance between destruction and reconstruction. Parathormone, calcitonin, local phosphate levels, thyroxine (T_4), and physical activity as well as the original inciting process modulate this process. Apparently some neoplasms, such as prostatic carcinoma, may produce factors that directly activate osteoblasts.

Two major factors—bone blood flow and bone turnover rates—have been identified as determining the degree of radiopharmaceutical uptake in bones on bone scans. Like most organs, bone in the resting state does not receive maximum blood flow, but approximately one-third of potential parallel blood flow

112

pathways through bone is closed by sympathetic tone. Processes that alter sympathetic tone affect bone blood flow, and therefore delivery of imaging agents to bone. The amount of mineral taken up by bone correlates with the metabolic state of the bone: cellular activation, collagen deposition, and mineral deposition. Chemiadsorption onto recently exposed or deposited bone crystal probably provides the chief mechanism of early mineral tracer uptake.

The major radiopharmaceuticals used for bone scans are the ^{99m}Tc-complexed organic and inorganic phosphate compounds, some with an added hydroxyl group to increase crystal binding. These include (1) pyrophosphate, which is simply two phosphate molecules linked together; (2) polyphosphate, a short chain of phosphate groups; and (3) diphosphonate compounds that have a P—C—P linkage binding replacing the P—O—P found in phosphates. The ^{99m}Tc diphosphonate compounds are most widely used for bone imaging because they have the most favorable blood clearance and bone uptake ratios. Approximately 50% of the injected dose is concentrated in the skeleton, and the remainder is excreted from the blood through the kidneys.

Radionuclide bone imaging is an extremely sensitive but nonspecific means of documenting localized sites of increased or decreased bone turnover. False-negative results occasionally occur. Clinically, radionuclide bone imaging has been valuable in detecting and following metastatic bone disease, as well as in evaluating bone trauma, vascular disorders, osteomyelitis, arthritis, and metabolic disease and in documenting ectopic bone formation. Nonspecific uptake of phosphate analogs also occurs in tissues undergoing cellular death, particularly muscle (e.g., acute myocardial infarction and skeletal muscle necrosis), and in sites of ectopic calcium deposition, such as the lungs in hyperparathyroidism.

NEOPLASMS

Studies show that 20–30% of bone metastases imaged on bone scans are missed on x-ray films. Approximately 5% of metastases may be evident on x-ray films of the bone, but not on bone scan. Particularly likely to escape detection by bone scan are those processes that infiltrate and replace marrow, such as multiple myeloma, reticulum cell sarcoma, leukemic processes, and histiocytosis X, rather than those that stimulate discrete bone resorption and production.

The role of bone scanning in evaluating patients with breast, lung, prostate (see Figs. 9-1 and 13-5, p. 169), and bowel cancers is discussed in Chapter 13. As a preoperative screening procedure in breast carcinoma, bone scanning remains controversial, but as a follow-up procedure and prognostic indicator this technique can be valuable. (See discussion in Chapter 13 on Specific Tumor Types and Adenocarcinoma of the Breast.) In bronchogenic carcinoma, for example, a true-positive bone scan indicates that survival for >1 year is unlikely. In prostate cancer, it is generally agreed that the bone scan is the most sensitive and effective screening test for metastases and is probably warranted in the preoperative staging of patients.

Although the bone scan has been used to follow the response of bone tumor lesions to chemotherapy, interpretation of these results must be guided by the knowledge that the bone scan is an indirect indication of the status of the tumor, since it only shows the effects of tumor on bone blood flow and bone turnover. Radiation induces changes in all tissues, including bone. Changes include vasculitis very early after irradiation, which may cause transient bone hyperemia followed by relative ischemia and diminution of osteoblastic cellular activity. These pathophysiologic consequences must be kept in mind when using the bone scan as a guide to following response of bone tumors to radiation therapy.

Benign bone neoplasms present bone scan images with varying degrees of radiopharmaceutical concentration. Typically, such lesions as osteoid osteomas, fibrous dysplasia, and Paget's disease are very hot (Fig. 9-2), whereas bone cysts, benign fibrous cortical defects, bone islands, eosinophilic granulomata, and most other benign bone lesions show either only mild degrees of increased uptake or normal uptake.

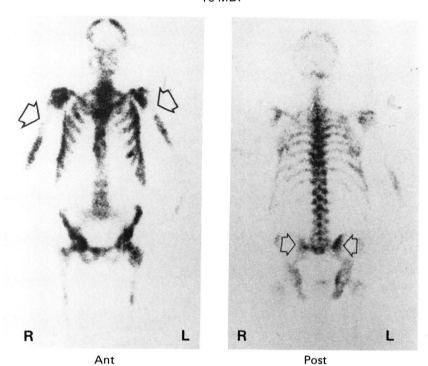

Fig. 9-1. Bone scan of patient with prostate cancer and widespread bone metastases performed on whole-body scanning scintillation camera. Images show markedly abnormal increased uptake of the ^{99m}Tc MDP distributed throughout the skeleton. Renal uptake is absent, and blood background activity is so low as to be nonimageable. This pattern is known as the superscan and indicates widespread bony disease. In addition to metastases, this pattern can be seen in metabolic bone disease, such as hyperparathyroidism. In metastatic disease, some region of asymmetry in the uptake is usually identifiable. Arrows indicate such regions of cold (photon-deficient) uptake in the humeri and asymmetry in the sacroiliac joints. Bone metastases manifest as either hot or cold foci on scans.

⁹⁹ᵐTc-HDP

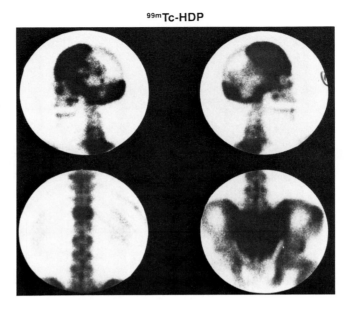

Fig. 9-2. Selected images from the bone scan of a patient with Paget's disease involving the skull, spine, and pelvis. Typically, because of the marked increase in bone blood flow and osteogenesis in Paget's disease, the bone scan shows marked augmentation in radiopharmaceutical uptake in affected bones. Bone scans have been found useful in assessing response to therapy and determining true activity of the disease in the patients.

TRAUMA

As many as 80% of patients with fractures have positive bone scans within 24 hr after fracture, and 95% of patients show positive findings by 72 hr. Sometimes, general diffuse uptake may occur reflecting loss of sympathetic tone with consequent increased tracer delivery. A radionuclide angiogram demonstrates this finding. With time, a more discrete deposition about the fracture site develops. Some fractures may be very difficult to visualize on x-ray film, particularly in the wrist, foot, face, and base of the skull, but easily seen on bone scan.

Fatigue or stress fractures are another category of bone

trauma that may not be evident on x-ray film, particularly at the time of onset of symptoms, but may be obvious on the bone scan (see Fig. 11-3, p. 144). Shin splints, which produce changes at the site of tibial muscle insertions, and may have a component of periosteal injury, but do not represent fracture, also have a characteristic bone scan appearance. They may show no changes on x-ray film. Failure of augmented radiopharmaceutical deposition in a fracture site weeks after the trauma suggests lack of an appropriate reparative response as, for example, in fibrous union. For additional discussion of bone scans in bone trauma, see Chapter 11.

VASCULAR DISEASE

Bone infarcts, particularly in patients with sickle cell disease, if imaged within the first few hours of onset, show characteristic focal absence of tracer. Within a day, however, nonspecific increased uptake apparently related to collateral circulation and bone repair can be seen, so that a bone scan performed at this time often cannot distinguish between infarction and infection.

Vascular disorders such as aseptic necrosis in the hips can be identified as deficient tracer uptake during early stages, before x-ray changes. Later during the remodeling and repair stage, augmented tracer uptake reflects the increased bone turnover of the reparative response. Particularly in elderly patients, the question of an avascular femoral head after hip fracture frequently arises. Bone scanning with a ^{99m}Tc-labeled phosphate compound combined with bone marrow imaging using ^{99m}Tc colloid, which localizes in the reticuloendothelial cells reflecting the status of the vascular integrity to the marrow in the femoral neck, may provide helpful data in predicting viability of the femoral head.

INFECTION

Osteomyelitis is usually evident on the bone scan early, 1 week to 10 days before x-ray changes become evident on x-ray films. Particularly in infants, the bone scan occasionally fails to show an abnormality, and radiopharmaceutical uptake may be normal. In this situation, the use of ^{67}Ga citrate as an indicator of inflammatory cell activity may be more sensitive and specific (see Chapter 12). Early in the pathophysiology of osteomyelitis, an infarction process may be caused by the infection and inflammation. This impairment of bone blood flow may be seen on the bone scan as a photon-deficient focus early in osteomyelitis, particularly in young children.

A very difficult clinical problem is differentiation of soft tissue infection from osteomyelitis (see Fig. 12-1, p. 153), particularly in diabetics and patients with peripheral vascular disease and nonhealing ulcers. Modification of the routine bone scan to a three-phase or four-phase bone scan which in addition to the routine static images also includes a radionuclide angiogram, blood-pool image, and multiple delayed images up to 24 hr post-injection aids the ability to distinguish between cellulitis and osteomyelitis (Fig. 9-3). Early images measure regional hyperemia. Delayed images identify uptake of tracer independent of hyperemia. Osteomyelitis demonstrates increasing lesion to background activity with time, whereas cellulitis shows the opposite.

METABOLIC DISEASE

Metabolic bone diseases, including Paget's disease, renal osteodystrophies, osteomalacia, osteoporosis, and hyperparathyroidism, may be detected and quantitated by bone scanning if computer analyses or urine collection counts, or both, are obtained. Response of the disease process to therapy may be documented objectively through serial bone scans. Complications of the disease such as insufficiency fractures, which result from normal stresses applied to abnormal bone, will also be evident on the bone scan.

JOINT DISEASE

In arthritis, increased joint activity is evident on the bone scan, particularly when active inflammation is present, stimulating

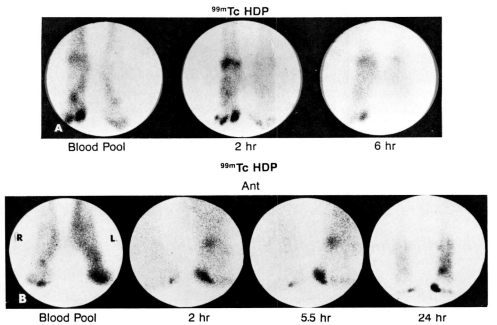

Fig. 9-3. (A) Blood-pool and 2- and 6-hr delayed images of the feet of a diabetic patient with an ulceration over the right great toe are shown. Hypervascularity to the right foot, particularly to the great toe, is evident on the blood-pool image. At 6 hr the activity shows a decreasing pattern reflecting cellulitis, with drainage of the ^{99m}Tc HDP from the lesion, similar to blood background behavior. **(B)** Blood-pool, 2-, 5.5-, and 24-hr delayed images of the feet of another diabetic patient with an ulceration over the left great toe are shown. Hypervascularity to the left foot, particularly the great toe, is evident. However, in this case, the abnormal increased activity over the left great toe does not decrease with time; it increases relative to blood background activity, reflecting osteomyelitis.

augmented blood flow to the joint and osteogenesis as a reaction of adjacent bony structures. These changes can be quantitated on the bone scan and response to therapy documented. The superior sensitivity of the bone scan over plain and weight-bearing x-ray films and arthrograms has been documented in reports on osteoarthritic degenerative disease, rheumatoid, and rheumatoid variant arthritides. The radiographic changes are, however, far more specific than the bone scan changes.

Septic arthritis is usually sensitively visualized on the bone scan. Determining whether the infection also involves the adjacent bones may be difficult. A bone marrow scan may be useful, as it should be normal unless osteomyelitis is present. In-111 leukocyte or Ga-67 scans may also be useful in such cases.

SOFT TISSUE LESIONS

Just as bone scanning agents are concentrated in regions of myocardial infarction (see discussion in Chapter 4), damaged muscle cells elsewhere and other calcified and noncalcified soft tissue lesions also concentrate the ^{99m}Tc-labeled phosphates (Fig. 9-4).

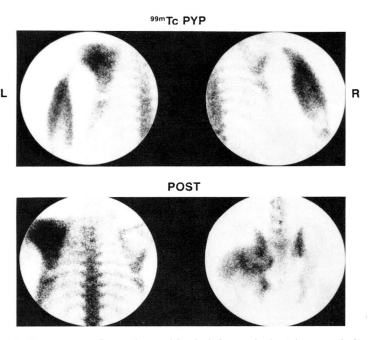

FIG. 9-4. Bone scan of a patient with rhabdomyolysis. Discrete skeletal muscle uptake of the ^{99m}Tc pyrophosphate is seen in muscles of the upper extremities, left gluteus, and left subscapularis.

The following are some examples of soft tissue lesions that may be visualized on bone scans: breast tumors, lactation, myocardial infarction, unstable angina, aneurysms, contusions of myocardial and skeletal muscle, calcified valves and arteries, amyloidosis, pericarditis, intestinal infarction, necrotizing enterocolitis, cerebral infarction, liver metastases, polymyositis, rhabdomyolysis, and myositis ossificans. Bone-forming tumors and those that calcify, such as neuroblastoma, osteosarcoma, colon cancer metastases, metastatic calcification, and diffuse interstitial pulmonary calcification, also concentrate the bone-seeking radiopharmaceuticals.

Ectopic ossification is well visualized on bone scans and is important to recognize as a possible postsurgical complication, sometimes seen in patients with hip prostheses. Another type of heterotopic para-articular ossification is noted in 20–30% of patients with spinal cord injury. During early stages of such formations, the bone scan shows striking uptake, reflecting the high degree of forming ossification and the immaturity of that ossification. As the ossification matures, the augmented ^{99m}Tc phosphate concentration diminishes until the degree of uptake stabilizes at a level comparable to that of mature bone. A bone marrow scan using ^{99m}Tc colloid demonstrates presence of bone marrow in the heterotopic bone when it has reached a mature state. At that time, rather than earlier, surgical removal of the heterotopic bone mass can be performed to relieve the immobilizing flexion deformity caused by the soft tissue ossification. Surgical excision attempted before maturity of the heterotopic ossification mass has a much higher incidence of recurrence than when mature heterotopic bone is removed.

SELECTED READINGS

Alazraki N. Bone imaging by radionuclide techniques. In: Resnick D, Niwayama A, eds. *Diagnosis of bone and joint disorders.* 2nd ed. Philadelphia: WB Saunders; 1988:460–505

Fogelman I (ed). *Bone scanning in clinical practice.* New York: Springer-Verlag; 1986

Howie DW, Savage JP, Wilson TG, et al. Technetium phosphate bone scan in the diagnosis of childhood osteomyelitis. *J Bone Joint Surg* 1983; 64A:431–437

Lull RJ, Utz JA, Jackson JH, et al. Radionuclide evaluation of joint disease. In: Freeman LM, Weissman HS, eds. *Nuclear medicine annual 1983*. New York: Raven Press; 1983:281–328

Matin P. Bone scans of trauma and benign conditions. In: Freeman LM, Weissmann HS, eds. *Nuclear medicine annual 1982*. New York: Raven Press; 1982:81–118

Matin P. The appearance of bone scans following fractures including immediate and long term studies. *J Nucl Med* 1979; 20:1227–1231

McDougall IR. Skeletal scintigraphy. *West J Med* 1979; 130:503–514

Rosenthall L, Lisbona R. *Skeletal imaging*. Norwalk, Conn: Appleton-Century-Crofts; 1984

Silberstein EB (ed). *Bone scintigraphy*. Mount Kisco, NY: Futura; 1984

Turner JH. Post-traumatic avascular necrosis of the femoral head predicted by preoperative technetium-99m antimony-colloid scan. *J Bone Joint Surg* 1983; 65A:786–797

10

Central Nervous System

Radiographic computed tomographic (CT) brain imaging and magnetic resonance imaging (MRI), because of their high sensitivity and ability to provide exquisite anatomic detail, are the imaging methods of choice in searching for brain lesions. Magnetic resonance imaging (MRI), now becoming more widely available, provides similar, and often better detail than CT and distinguishes parenchymal gray and white matter lesions with greater sensitivity than CT. Conventional blood-brain-barrier radionuclide brain imaging is rarely used now. MRI and CT scanning have superior sensitivity in detecting most intracranial lesions. Both MRI and the CT scan give details of brain anatomy not seen on the radionuclide scan. The radionuclide cerebral angiogram shows relative cerebral perfusion, and the conventional brain scan reflects the integrity of the blood-brain barrier. The development of positron and single photon emitting tracers of brain blood flow and metabolism promise to provide unique means for understanding normal and abnormal brain function. They also provide sensitive means for detecting functional brain abnormalities.

PET IMAGING

Functional images of regional brain metabolism and blood flow using positron emission tomography (PET) techniques have been achieved in normal and diseased states. As an example, fluorine-

123

18-labeled fluorodeoxyglucose (^{18}F FDG) is taken into brain cells in the same way as glucose but, because it cannot be metabolized after phosphorylation, it remains relatively fixed in these cells as it was deposited. PET images of the distribution of ^{18}F FDG therefore reflect regional glucose utilization.

PET can detect abnormalities not apparent by other modalities. In Huntington's disease, for example, reduced caudate nucleus glucose metabolism has been seen on PET images in asymptomatic individuals identified by chromosomal analysis as being at risk for the disease. Characteristic image patterns have been identified on the PET studies of subjects with dementia of the Alzheimer type, which permit their distinction from other dementias. Figure 10-1 shows ^{18}F FDG PET brain images in a depressed patient and in patients with multi-infarct dementia and with dementia of the Alzheimer type. Foci of cortical or subcortical sites responsible for triggering seizures in epileptic patients can also be identified by PET imaging. Brain tumor recurrence may be distinguished from radiation necrosis using ^{11}C-labeled amino acids which are taken up in recurrent tumor but not in areas of radiation necrosis where there is little or no protein synthesis.

PET imaging of neuroreceptors provides a fascinating new insight into brain function in health and disease. Thus far, the dopaminergic sites have been visualized using labeled spiperone, the cholinergic sites using quinuclidinyl benzilate (QNB) derivatives, and the opiate receptors using labeled carfentinil. By spatially localizing and quantifying neuroreceptor sites, PET studies permit identification of loss of neuroreceptors in disease states and provide a means of objectively quantifying saturation of neuroreceptor sites by various therapeutic regimens. This approach adds a new dimension to the exploration of brain disease and will undoubtedly give us pathophysiologic insights that were not possible in the living brain with other techniques. Such an understanding is the first step to objective diagnosis and eventual development of appropriate therapy.

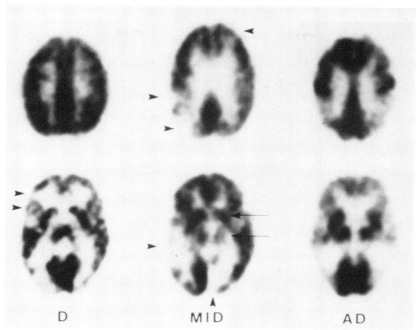

FIG. 10-1. PET studies of regional cerebral glucose utilization using ^{18}F-labeled fluorodeoxyglucose as an indicator of metabolic activity. Transverse sections at two different levels from a patient with depression **(D)** show high cortical gray matter activity in a symmetric fashion with slight decrease in the right frontal region (*arrows*) found in depression. Little activity is seen in the white matter, whereas the thalamus and caudate nucleus are readily apparent. Transverse sections from two levels of the brain in a patient with multi-infarct dementia **(MID)** show multiple areas of reduced glucose utilization scattered throughout the cortex as well as the basal ganglia (*arrows*). Transverse sections from two levels of the brain in a patient with dementia of the Alzheimer type **(AD)**. Symmetric decrease in glucose metabolism is apparent in the parietal regions. The basal ganglia and thalamus can be seen as central structures with metabolic activity approximating that of normal cortical gray matter, while the less metabolically active white matter is seen as clear areas of low metabolic activity. (Reprinted from Kuhl DE: *Radiology* 1984; 150:625–631, by permission of the author and the Radiological Society of North America.)

SPECT IMAGING

The recent introduction of the lipophilic technetium-labeled cerebral blood flow agent ^{99m}Tc *dl*-hexamethylpropyleneamine oxime (HMPAO) imaged with single-photon emission computed tomography (SPECT) provides a clinical tool for estimating regional cerebral blood flow. Although still investigational, this compound will eventually be readily available in kit form. Unlike the positron indicators of blood flow, this compound remains relatively fixed intracellularly after a small initial redistribution. In ischemic stroke, the SPECT HMPAO brain scan shows immediate evidence of decreased blood flow that is not evident on purely anatomic studies such as CT or MRI. Figure 10-2 shows the appearance of transverse plane cross-sectional images in a

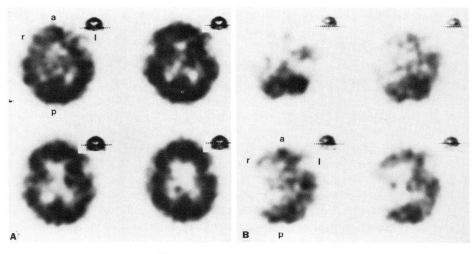

FIG. 10-2. (A) Normal ^{99m}Tc HMPAO SPECT images of the brain from base of brain toward the vertex show activity uniformly outlining cortical blood flow with visualization of the basal ganglia. Small superimposed images with dotted lines indicate level of section as seen in frontal projection. **(B)** Patient with large right hemispheric infarction resulting in left hemiplegia and aphasia shows marked decrease in blood flow to the right cerebral hemisphere on the ^{99m}Tc HMPAO SPECT study. (Cases courtesy of Richard A Holmes, M.D., Professor of Radiology and Medicine, University of Missouri, Harry S. Truman Memorial Veterans Hospital, Columbia, Missouri.)

normal individual and in a patient with an acute large ischemic infarct of the right cerebral hemisphere.

Because ^{99m}Tc HMPAO does not redistribute with time, it can be used to indicate evanescent cerebral blood flow changes occurring for only a brief duration. For example, ^{99m}Tc HMPAO can be injected during a state of mental activity or induced cortical stimulation, drug administration, or even the occurrence of a seizure. Imaging even 1–2 hr later will reflect the cerebral blood flow at the time of tracer injection rather than at the time of imaging. This technique provides a powerful tool for studying regional transient increase or decrease in brain blood flow.

Similar results in ischemic brain disease have been obtained with SPECT imaging of ^{123}I-labeled amines, including N-isopropyl ^{123}I iodoamphetamine (^{123}I IMP) and ^{123}I-labeled HIPDM. These agents undergo redistribution with time and, although the initial delivery is via blood flow, their cellular uptake reflects brain cell metabolic activity. Uncoupling of blood flow and metabolic activity may take place in ischemic brain tissue when vessels become patent, while the tissue they supply has undergone irreversible change following the ischemic episode. Such uncoupling of blood flow from cellular metabolic activity occurs in the luxury perfusion syndrome in which blood flow exceeding tissue metabolic requirements follows an ischemic episode.

RADIONUCLIDE CEREBRAL ANGIOGRAPHY

Vascular Problems

Immediately after a peripheral intravenous (i.v.) injection of a ^{99m}Tc radiopharmaceutical such as ^{99m}Tc DTPA for brain imaging, a radionuclide cerebral angiogram can be obtained that shows relative perfusion between the two hemispheres as well as the relative rates of appearance of the radiopharmaceutical in neck vessels. The neck vessels are seen as the superimposition of the carotid and vertebral vessels, and only severe vascular obstructions will be evident. Highly vascular lesions in the brain will be obvious as regions of focally increased activity; for example, arteriovenous (AV) malformations and vascular tumors such as the meningioma and glioblastoma multiforme are easily identified.

Focal regions of decreased radiopharmaceutical perfusion may be evident in patients with vascular problems, such as cerebrovascular accidents (CVAs) (Fig. 10-3A) and subdural hematomas or masses large enough to compress the brain significantly and reduce perfusion. Typically, in patients who have sustained a recent stroke, the radionuclide angiogram shows a flip-flop of activity. Flip-flop describes the sequence of diminished perfusion during the arterial phase transforming to augmented tracer activity during the later venous phase of the radionuclide angiogram. This phenomenon is explained as initial slowed and reduced perfusion to the affected region, followed by delayed arrival and increased transit time of radiopharmaceutical through collaterals, resulting in relative increased activity in the affected region after the normal side has drained its activity.

Occasionally the radionuclide cerebral angiogram shows locally increased perfusion in ischemic lesions, as in some patients with recent infarction, trauma, and prolonged seizures. The hyperemia is believed to result from lactic acidosis of hypoxic tissues that provokes localized dilation of the arteriolar bed. Because the damaged cerebral tissue fails to extract most of the oxygen brought to it, the venous blood emerging from the area has a relatively high oxygen content and appears red, like arterial blood. Failure of complete extraction of oxygen implies that the region is receiving blood in excess of its metabolic needs, constituting a luxury perfusion syndrome.

Cerebral Death

Cerebral death is manifested as absence of cerebral perfusion on the radionuclide angiogram. Increased cerebral tissue pressure, if generalized as in severe edema, shuts off capillary perfusion and ultimately cuts off arterial blood flow to the brain, leading to

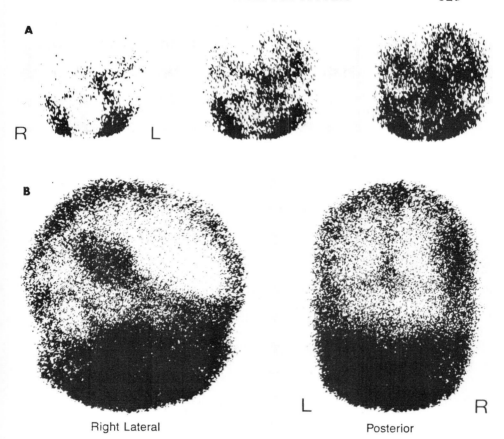

Right Lateral

Posterior

FIG. 10-3. **(A)** Radionuclide cerebral angiogram performed in the anterior view, with the scintillation camera positioned over the head. Selected images accumulated at 3 sec per frame show impaired perfusion of the right hemisphere in a 55-yr-old patient who had a right-sided cerebral infarct secondary to embolus. **(B)** Brain scan. Right lateral and posterior projections in the same patient shown in **A**. The brain scan images show focal increased uptake in the distribution of the posterior parietal and angular branches of the right middle cerebral artery, consistent with infarction. The tracer used was ^{99m}Tc glucoheptonate.

cellular death. The radionuclide angiogram in cerebral death shows activity circulating only through the arteries of the face and external carotid arteries, with absent perfusion in the regions corresponding to the middle and anterior cerebral arteries; there is no visualization of the sagittal sinus. In the case of cerebral death that has been present for a day or two, the blood-brain barrier shows general disruption, and activity may leak into the brain from the periphery. Brain death invariably follows cerebral death.

DELAYED BRAIN SCAN IMAGES

Focal Lesions

Approximately 2 hr after i.v. injection of the radiopharmaceutical, delayed static images are obtained over the head in several projections. These images make up the conventional radionuclide blood-brain-barrier brain scan, showing the distribution of the radiopharmaceutical in the normal vascular spaces and facial structures. Brain tissue excludes the radiopharmaceutical and is imaged normally as low background activity. Thus, the normal brain and its anatomic details cannot be seen on a brain scan. In the presence of an abnormality, such as infarct (Fig. 10-3B), neoplasm (Fig. 10-4), abscess, hematoma, or other lesion disturbing the normal blood-brain barrier, the radiopharmaceutical is concentrated in the abnormal region, because of the disruption of the normal blood-brain barrier, perhaps related to the effect of the lesion on capillary permeability.

In herpes simplex encephalitis—the most common form of sporadic encephalitis—the radionuclide study is abnormal very early in the course of the disease, showing marked focal hyperemia and breakdown of the blood-brain barrier typically in the temporoparietal region. In other forms of encephalitis and in diffuse meningitis, the brain scan may show a diffuse abnormal uptake, but often appears totally normal. Occasionally, focal abnormalities may be seen.

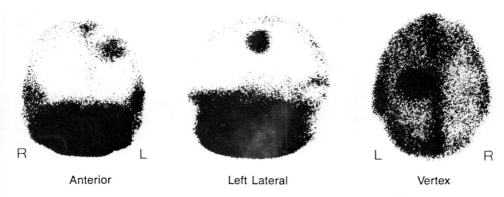

Anterior   Left Lateral   Vertex

FIG. 10-4. Brain scan. Two hours after i.v. injection of ^{99m}Tc glucoheptonate, images over the head were made in multiple projections. The anterior, left lateral, and vertex views are shown. A focal region of well-defined increased activity is seen in the left parietal region. The finding is consistent with primary brain tumor or a metastatic brain lesion. Abscess, hematoma, or any localized abnormality causing disruption of the blood-brain barrier or replacing normal cerebral tissue could cause a similar abnormality on brain scan. In this case, the lesion was a metastatic adenocarcinoma from the lung.

Laminar cortical necrosis caused by a brief anoxic or metabolic insult such as hypoglycemia shows a diffuse peripheral cortical uptake pattern.

Effects of Therapy

Systemic corticosteroids may reduce or eliminate focal uptake related to cerebral tumors. Radiation therapy also alters the uptake of the radiopharmaceutical by brain lesions. Immediately after delivery of 35–60 Gy (3500–6000 rad), increased tracer uptake may be seen in a tumor, reflecting a hypervascular response to the radiation. Much later, decreased uptake may be observed, reflecting tissue damage or reappearance of the initial level of abnormal uptake may be seen. Imaging with thallium-201 may be helpful in such cases, since it is taken up in sites of viable tumor, but not in radiation necrosis.

CEREBROSPINAL FLUID DYNAMICS

Radionuclide Cisternography

Radionuclide cisternography provides images of the distribution and movement of cerebrospinal fluid (CSF) after the intrathecal administration of a radiopharmaceutical (see discussion below), usually at the L4–5 level. Radiopharmaceutical administration by a "hyperbaric" technique uses 10% dextrose in water to carry the radiopharmaceutical cephalad with the patient in Trendelenburg position. This procedure minimizes leakage at the injection site and decreases the percentage of technical failures. Soon after moving cephalad from the injection site, the hypertonicity of the 10% dextrose is lost; bulk movement of isotonic materials is not influenced by patient position.

Imaging is performed over the spine and over the head in multiple projections at 4, 24, 48, and 72 hr as necessary after intrathecal administration of the radiopharmaceutical. Normally the tracer ascends to the head and flows into the cisterna magna, the basal cisterns, the Sylvian fissure spaces, posteriorly to the ambiens cisterns and quadrigeminal cisterns, and over the convexities to the subarachnoid granulations, where resorption into the blood occurs. If the tracer penetrates the ventricular system and persists there for 24 hr, abnormal CSF dynamics and probably hydrocephalus are present (Fig. 10-5). MRI or radiographic CT scanning easily identifies ventricular dilatation. Radionuclide cisternography defines the pathways of CSF flow.

Rates of production and resorption of CSF vary with patient age. Children have more rapid turnover of CSF than do adults. In normal adults, CSF is produced at a rate of ~0.35 ml/min, an amount commensurate with total CSF turnover four times per 24 hr. On the radionuclide cisternogram, comparing counts in the brain on a 24-hr image with a 48-hr image, and correcting for decay of the radionuclide, the disappearance of tracer through resorption into the blood can be calculated. The normal half-time disappearance of CSF in the head on the cisternogram varies from ~12 hr in younger patients to ~24–48 hr in older patients.

¹¹¹In DTPA Cisternogram

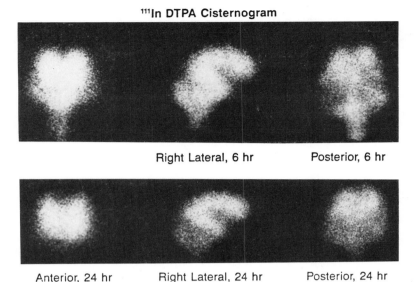

Right Lateral, 6 hr   Posterior, 6 hr

Anterior, 24 hr   Right Lateral, 24 hr   Posterior, 24 hr

FIG. 10-5. Indium-111 DTPA cisternogram images at 6 hr and 24 hr after intrathecal administration of the radiopharmaceutical. Anterior, right lateral, and posterior views show enlarged ventricles with persistent activity in the ventricles at 24 hr and poor flow of tracer in cerebrospinal fluid (CSF) over the convexities. Analysis of count-time data from the images shows poor resorption of the radiopharmaceutical from the CSF. These findings are consistent with normal-pressure hydrocephalus.

This differs significantly from the known CSF production and turnover data because in performing cisternography, the radiopharmaceutical is injected at one point in the CSF, from which it moves by bulk flow and hence never truly attains an even distribution.

Normal-Pressure Hydrocephalus: The findings on the radionuclide cisternogram in patients with normal-pressure hydrocephalus include persistence of activity in the ventricles with ventricular enlargement, slowed flow and paucity of tracer above the convexities, and delayed resorption of the radiopharmaceutical at the subarachnoid granulations (Fig. 10-5). If slowed resorption of radiopharmaceutical, and presumably CSF as well, is identified, and if ventricular penetration and persistence of the radiopharmaceutical within the ventricular system are identified, the patient may benefit from a surgical shunt to remove CSF from the ventricles. Unfortunately, clinical follow-up of patients treated with shunts does not seem to correlate well with such findings. Rather, duration of symptoms before shunting seems to correlate best with clinical response to surgical shunt procedures. Patients operated on within 6 mo of onset of symptoms are more likely to show clinical improvement in their symptoms than are those who have been symptomatic for more than 6 mo before undergoing shunt placement.

CSF Leaks and Shunts: Other problems in CSF dynamics that can be detected and sometimes quantitated by radionuclide cisternography include CSF rhinorrhea or otorrhea and de- termination of patency of diversionary shunts. In the evaluation of CSF leaks, if there is sufficient fluid leakage, images can demonstrate the leaking fluid after intrathecal administration of the radiopharmaceutical. In the absence of image identification of the leak, carefully weighed cotton pledgets are placed in the nasal cavities or ear canals and are counted 4–6 hr later. If a ratio >1.5 of counts, expressed as counts per gram, is found in the pledgets relative to counts per milliliter in plasma, CSF leakage is confirmed.

Radiopharmaceuticals for Cisternography: Ideally, the radiopharmaceutical should be of sufficiently low molecular weight so that it can be carried by CSF bulk flow, but of a large enough molecular size so that it is not absorbed into blood through surrounding arachnoidal blood capillaries. The physical half-life of the radionuclide should be long enough to permit imaging as late as 72 hr, and the biologic half-life should be short enough to minimize radiation exposure. The materials must be nontoxic and pyrogen free and should have a γ-ray energy suit- able for imaging. The most widely used radiopharmaceutical is ^{111}In DTPA. Technetium-99m DTPA can be used for diversionary shunt patency studies and cisternograms in children, but the 6-hr physical half-life of ^{99m}Tc makes it unsuitable for radionuclide cisternograms in adults.

SELECTED READINGS

Alazraki NP, Halpern SE, Ashburn WL, et al. Hyperbaric cisternography: Experience in humans. *J Nucl Med* 1973; 14(4):226–229

Front D. Current practice in nuclear medicine. In: Baum S, ed. *Radionuclide brain imaging.* East Norwalk, CT: Appleton & Lange; 1982:1–141

Frost JJ, Wagner HN Jr, Dannals RF, et al. Imaging opiate receptors in the human brain by positron tomography. *J Comput Assist Tomogr* 1985; 9:231–236

Harbert JC, Rocha AF. The central nervous system. In: Rocha AF, Harbert JC, eds. *Textbook of nuclear medicine: Clinical applications.* Philadelphia: Lea & Febiger; 1979:51–108

Holman BL, Gibson RE, Hill TC, et al. Muscarinic acetylcholine receptors in Alzheimer's disease. In vivo imaging with iodine 123-labeled 3-quinuclidinyl-4-iodobenzilate and emission tomography. *JAMA* 1985; 254:3063–3066

Magistretti PL (ed). *Functional radionuclide imaging of the brain.* New York: Raven Press; 1983:1–368

Mazziotta JC, Phelps ME, Pahl JJ, et al. Reduced glucose metabolism in asymptomatic subjects at risk for Huntington's disease. *N Engl J Med* 1987; 316:357–62

Mishkin FS. Cerebral radionuclide angiography. *Angiology* 1977; 28:261–275

Neirinckx RD, Channing LR, Piper IM, et al. Technetium-99m d,-HMPAO: A new radiopharmaceutical for SPECT imaging of regional cerebral blood perfusion. *J Nucl Med* 1987; 28:191–202

Phelps ME, Mazziotta JC, Huang SC. Study of cerebral function with positron computed tomography. *J Cereb Blood Flow Metab* 1982; 2:113–162

Research issues in positron emission tomography. *Proceedings of a conference of the National Institute of Neurological and Communicative Disorders and Stroke.* Bethesda, MD: National Institutes of Health; 1984

Siegel BA (ed). *Nuclear radiology syllabus*, Ser. 2. Chicago: American College of Radiology; 1978:192–255

Wagner HN Jr. Probing the chemistry of the mind. *N Engl J Med* 1985; 312:44–46

Wagner HN Jr, Burns HD, Dannals RF, et al. Imaging dopamine receptors in the human brain by positron tomography. *Science* 1983; 221:1264–1266

Imaging Disease Processes

11
Trauma

Evaluation of traumatized patients by radionuclide scintigraphy offers the advantages of safety, simplicity, sensitivity, and usually ready availability. The radionuclide study may be used as a screening procedure to help determine the need for, or appropriateness of, a more invasive radiographic or surgical procedure. It can also be used to substantiate a diagnosis. Additional comments on bone trauma may also be found in Chapter 9.

BRAIN

The most common serious complication of head trauma referred for diagnostic imaging studies is subdural hematoma (SDH). Acute and subacute SDH are best diagnosed by MRI or computed tomography (CT) scanning, where this is available. A radionuclide angiogram involving sequential images of the head at approximately every 2 sec for ~1 min after the intravenous (i.v.) injection of a radiopharmaceutical will demonstrate a persistently avascular area in the region of the hematoma if it is sufficiently large. In ~80% of cases of chronic SDH and, to a lesser degree in the subacute phase, delayed images of the brain at 2 hr after injection will show increased uptake in the region of a hematoma on anterior or posterior views, or both. In acute SDH, the characteristic abnormal pattern on the radionuclide angiogram and normal static images are usually seen.

In patients suspected of epidural collection, delay for the nonspecific radionuclide exam only impedes prompt therapeutic intervention. Computed tomography (CT) or contrast angiography should be performed immediately in these patients.

139

A radionuclide angiogram after a peripheral intravenous bolus injection reliably identifies the presence or absence of cerebral perfusion, and hence cerebral death (see Chapter 10).

LIVER

Iatrogenic trauma from closed liver biopsy producing subcapsular or intrahepatic hematomas seldom requires surgical intervention. However, surgical intervention may be needed for penetrating wounds, especially when there is leakage of blood or bile into the peritoneal cavity or retroperitoneum.

A radionuclide angiogram using intravenously injected ^{99m}Tc colloid, followed by images of the liver in multiple projections, may provide evidence of blood leakage and identify its source, while ^{99m}Tc IDA (see Chapter 7) will demonstrate biliary leaks in patients who have had biliary surgery or a penetrating abdominal wound. The radionuclide liver image is quite sensitive in detecting clinically significant hepatic lacerations or hematomas. In most institutions equipped with CT, that modality is the first-line diagnostic tool in cases of abdominal trauma. Abdominal CT scans show abnormalities of the liver, spleen, pancreas, kidneys, and gastrointestinal tract. However, a specific nuclear medicine study is often useful in pinpointing the areas of concern for imaging with CT or ultrasound.

SPLEEN

After blunt abdominal trauma, left upper quadrant pain, with or without evidence of intra-abdominal blood loss, may reflect a fractured spleen. A radionuclide angiogram using ^{99m}Tc colloid followed by static images may show a fractured spleen or intrasplenic hematoma as a focus of decreased counts (Fig. 11-1).

The diagnosis of splenic trauma is fraught with pitfalls, however. Many normal variants of splenic morphology exist, hence caution is necessary in interpretation. Lobulations may mimic fracture lines, and variations such as "hooked" spleen and indentation by a distended stomach may have the appearance of

Tc-99m Colloid

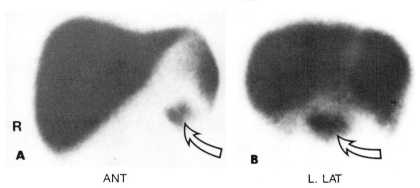

ANT   L. LAT

FIG. 11-1. Splenic rupture in a 6-yr-old boy struck by a car. (**A**) Anterior view shows functioning fragment of spleen beneath the main splenic mass (*arrow*). (**B**) Confirmed on the left lateral view (*arrow*).

hematoma or other splenic lesions. Sensitivity is probably better than 95%, but specificity is only moderate. The occurrence of false-positive studies makes angiography preferable before surgery. Spleen scans provide a convenient means of following conservative management of children with ruptured spleens. The use of ^{99m}Tc heat-damaged red blood cells instead of ^{99m}Tc colloid confines the uptake to splenic tissue, eliminating visualization of the liver on images. This may be helpful if there is liver enlargement or overlap with splenic tissue.

KIDNEY

Blunt abdominal trauma or penetrating wounds may produce fracture of the kidney or intrarenal abnormalities. Static images after i.v. injection of ^{99m}Tc glucoheptonate, ^{99m}Tc DTPA, or ^{99m}Tc dimercaptosuccinic acid (DMSA) will demonstrate morphologic disruptions. Combined with a radionuclide angiogram, these imaging studies can evaluate the vascular supply to the kidney, the integrity of the organ, and its functional state. Urinary leakage and the presence of accumulating urinomas may be identified either by technetium studies or by using labeled ^{131}I orthoiodohippurate (hippuran). Similarly, imaging over the pelvis may show evidence of trauma to the bladder either by leakage of the radiopharmaceutical or by deformity resulting from hematomas. The sensitivity of the appropriate radionuclide study in detecting abnormalities requiring surgical intervention is high.

VASCULAR

After penetrating wounds of the extremities, abdomen, or chest, a hematoma or bleeding from a large vessel and the presence or absence of a pseudoaneurysm may be a clinical concern. An angiographic study with any of the commonly used ^{99m}Tc-labeled agents may demonstrate the presence of these lesions, although not with the certainty and anatomic preciseness of an intra-arterial catheter-contrast injection or an i.v. digital subtraction radiographic angiogram required for surgical intervention. The sensitivity in detecting abnormalities in large limb vessels is about the same as that in contrast angiography.

BONE

In contrast to rib metastases, which are usually haphazardly located, rib fractures often show a characteristic pattern of a lineup of abnormal focal hot lesions in the ribs affected. Rib fractures seen on bone scan may be unsuspected after a fall, an automobile accident (steering wheel injury), or overenthusiastic cardiopulmonary resuscitation (CPR). Or, the patient may have exquisite pain at a costochondral junction site with no abnormality observed on x-ray film. The bone scan usually shows a focal hot region at this site of cartilage trauma (Fig. 11-2).

Stress fractures resulting from abnormal repetitive stress on normal bone may produce clinical pain, yet show no abnormal findings on x-ray film of the bone. Bone scans are able to show clear focal abnormalities (Fig. 11-3). Periosteal injuries that mimic stress fractures in their clinical presentation and lack of x-ray findings show a characteristic bone scan appearance.* An abnor-

---

*For a discussion of shin splint injuries, see Chapter 9.

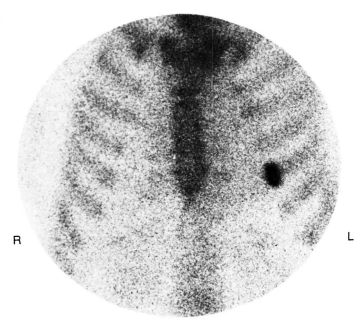

FIG. 11-2. Anterior view of the chest shows focal increased uptake at the costochondral junction of a left rib. Radiographs showed no fracture, but the patient had exquisite pain at this site of cartilage injury.

mal vertical pattern of increased uptake is seen along the injured bone, rather than horizontally crossing the width of the shaft, as in true stress fractures. Athletes with periosteal injuries can usually return to their activities in a few weeks, while stress fractures may require more time to heal.

Hairline fractures may also be difficult to document on routine radiography, especially in such areas as the mastoid, wrist, foot, or face, but are often easily seen on the bone scan. Where a collapsed vertebra is seen on the x-ray film, with or without trauma, the bone scan may be able to estimate the age of the fracture as recent versus old. In 95% of patients under age 65, the bone scan will demonstrate increased bone turnover within 48 hr of the traumatic event, and almost all patients will be found to have an abnormality by 72 hr. Lack of tracer uptake in a collapsed verebra means that recent fracture is unlikely to account for the collapse.

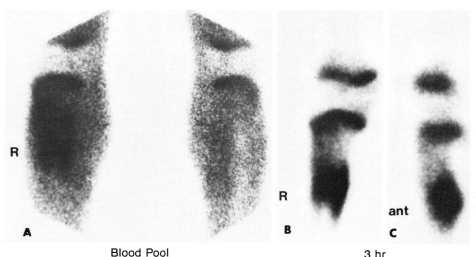

Blood Pool   3 hr

FIG. 11-3. Stress fracture affecting tibial cortex in a 15-yr-old jogger. (**A**) Blood-pool image of both knees immediately after injection of ^{99m}Tc MDP shows hyperemia of the proximal right tibia. (**B,C**) Anterior and lateral views (3 hr later), respectively, show marked increase in cortical uptake in the proximal tibia as well as normal epiphyseal uptake. The x-ray film, which was normal at the time of the bone scan, later showed reactive bone formation.

Some studies reported on evaluation of battered children for bone trauma have recommended whole-body radionuclide bone imaging plus x-ray films of the skull as suitable screening procedures. Others suggest x-ray skeletal surveys. In adults or children, when a fractured long bone appears to be healing poorly, or when a pseudoarthrosis is suspected, the ^{99m}TC phosphate bone scan can be used to evaluate the healing process and the presence of interruption in callus formation. The bone scan is also useful in predicting the success or failure of bone grafts as well as reimplantation of a severed limb.

Bone imaging provides a sensitive means of detecting changes accompanying meniscal tears in the knee, especially with the use of SPECT. MRI is probably the best available imaging modality for evaluating knee pain since meniscal tears, ligamentous tears, and bone as well as soft tissue injuries are exquisitely seen. Bone imaging provides only indirect evidence of cartilagenous damage through its effects on bone. Planar bone imaging and SPECT imaging can also aid in detecting the subtle changes of spondylolysis in the lumbar spine.

LUNG

In known lung trauma, lung scans can evaluate the extent of abnormally perfused and ventilated lung. Imaging following peripheral i.v. injection of ^{133}Xe dissolved in saline shows perfusion as well as ventilation and can document loss of integrity of the bronchial tree. In burn victims, an i.v. xenon study has been found to be sensitive for localizing and evaluating damage to the respiratory system.

SELECTED READINGS

General

Berg BC. Emergency applications of nuclear medicine. In Freeman LM, Weissmann HS, eds. *Nuclear medicine annual 1981.* New York: Raven Press, 1981:275–314

Berg BC. The use of radionuclide imaging in diagnosis management of the "acute" or traumatized patient. In: Gottschalk A, Potchen EJ, eds. *Diagnostic nuclear medicine.* Baltimore: Williams & Wilkins; 1976:550–563

Brain

Alderson PO, Gado MH, Siegel BA. Computerized cranial tomography and radionuclide imaging in the detection of intracranial mass lesions. *Semin Nucl Med* 1977; 7:161–173

Brown R, Weber PM, dos Remedios LV. Dynamic/static brain scintigraphy: An effective screening test for subdural hematoma. *Radiology* 1975; 117:355–360

Cowan RJ, Maynard CD. Trauma to the brain and extracranial structures. *Semin Nucl Med* 1974; 4:319–338

Goodman JM, Heck LR. Confirmation of brain death at bedside by isotope angiography. *JAMA* 1977; 238:966–968

Liver

Lutzker L. Radionuclide imaging of the injured spleen and liver. *Semin Nucl Med* 1983; 13:184–198

Spleen

Nebesar RA, Rabinov KR, Potsaid MS. Radionuclide imaging of the spleen in suspected splenic injury. *Radiology* 1974; 110:609–614

Kidney

Berg BC. Radionuclide studies after urinary tract injury. *Semin Nucl Med* 1974; 4:371–393

Vascular

Rudavsky AZ, Moss CM. Radionuclide angiography for the evaluation of peripheral vascular injuries. In: Freeman LM, Weissmann HS, eds. *Nuclear medicine annual 1981.* New York: Raven Press; 1981:315–335

Bone

Collier BD, Johnson RP, Carrera GF, et al. Chronic knee pain assessed by SPECT: Comparison with other modalities. *Radiology* 1985; 157:795–802

Marty R, Denney JD, McKamery MR, et al. Bone trauma and related benign disease: Assessment by bone scanning. *J Nucl Med* 1976; 6:107–120

Matin P. The appearance of bone scans following fractures, including immediate and long term studies. *J Nucl Med* 1979; 20:1227–1231

Matin P. Bone scintigraphy in the diagnosis and management of traumatic injury. *Semin Nucl Med* 1983; 13:104–122

Papanicolaou N, Wilkinson RH, Emans JE, et al. Bone scintigraphy and radiography in young athletes with low back pain. *AJR* 1985; 145:1039–1044

Lung

Lull RJ, Tatum JL, Sugarman HJ, et al. Radionuclide evaluation of lung trauma. *Semin Nucl Med* 1983; 13:223–237

12

Inflammatory and Infectious Processes

Selected radionuclide studies can serve as a sensitive screening method for detecting inflammatory or infectious processes. Organ imaging procedures, such as brain, liver, bone, and kidney scans, can detect an infectious focus; however, findings are nonspecific and can be seen in processes other than infection, including neoplasm, other masses, vascular impairment, or trauma. More direct approaches include the use of ^{67}Ga citrate, although it too is a nonspecific test, and ^{111}In-labeled polymorphonuclear leukocytes.

MULTIORGAN IMAGING

Liver–Spleen Scans

Technetium-99m sulfur colloid used in liver–spleen scans shows liver abscesses as focal lesions and may show subdiaphragmatic abscesses as impressions in the dome, posterior, or lateral aspect of the liver. Most subdiaphragmatic abscesses actually lie in the subhepatic space in the superior recess of the right suprarenal area known as Morison's pouch. These processes cause indentation of the posterior inferior hepatic margin adjacent to the renal bed. Tumors, cysts, hematomas, or loculated fluid can yield indistinguishable scan abnormalities. Gallium will concentrate in hepatic abscesses and neoplasms, but not in cysts, hematomas, or noninfected fluid collections; it can therefore be useful in

148

characterizing a liver scan abnormality. Indium-111-labeled leukocytes will also localize in hepatic abscesses, but not in cysts, hematomas, or noninfected fluid collections. Indium-111 leukocytes are much less likely than gallium to concentrate in tumors. With either agent, gallium or ^{111}In leukocytes, a conventional ^{99m}Tc liver–spleen scan must also be performed to identify the abnormal region, which is then characterized by how it handles gallium or ^{111}In leukocytes.

Renal Scintigraphy

Agents such as ^{99m}Tc-labeled glucoheptonate, DTPA, or DMSA used in renal scintigraphy will show focal abnormalities and usually diminished overall function in the kidney with pyelonephritis or abscess. The sensitivity for detecting such renal parenchymal processes may exceed that with excretory urography, but again the findings are nonspecific. Computed tomography, ultrasound, and gallium imaging add specificity. Gallium concentrates in active pyelonephritis, while normal kidneys imaged 72 hr after gallium injection usually show little uptake. Gallium imaging can help in distinguishing lower tract urinary infection from upper tract disease, or by diagnosing both.

Bone Scanning

Using ^{99m}Tc phosphates or diphosphonates, bone scanning is sensitive in detecting the increased bone blood flow and bone mineral turnover associated with osteomyelitis, localizing the disease process 1–2 wk before discernible radiographic changes take place. The three-phase or four-phase bone scan (see Fig. 9-3, p. 119) is useful in distinguishing between osteomyelitis and cellulitis, often a very difficult clinical problem (see discussion in Chapter 9). Again, many bony abnormalities provoke a similar bone response, including benign or malignant neoplasms, infarct repair, trauma, and postsurgical changes. Occasionally, particularly in neonates and small children, acute osteomyelitis imaged early appears as an area of diminished uptake, presumably related to ischemia and infarction produced by inflammatory cells infiltrating the marrow spaces and sinusoids. Compared with results in adults, a higher incidence of false-negative bone scans is reported in neonates with early osteomyelitis; therefore, in this group a normal bone scan does not exclude bone infection (see also Chapter 9). A gallium scan, reserved as a second line diagnostic imaging test because of the higher radiation dose associated with its use, may be required in neonates and young children suspected of having osteomyelitis if the bone scan is normal. MRI can be very helpful.

Radionuclide Brain Scanning

Technetium-99m pertechnetate, glucoheptonate, or DTPA can detect >90% of cerebral abscesses as well as the earlier stages of cerebritis. Again, the increased activity attributable to the blood-brain barrier deficit provoked in the brain by infection occurs with many other pathologic processes.

GALLIUM-67 IMAGING

Gallium-67 citrate imaging is widely used as a screening procedure in detecting sites of infection. After intravenous injection, ^{67}Ga citrate, a group IIIB metal, is carried in the blood bound to transferrin and other proteins. Gallium is accumulated in normal tissues, including the liver, spleen, bone marrow, nasopharynx, lacrimal glands, and the prolactin-stimulated or lactating breast. Renal excretion is highest during the first 24 hr; later, excretion by colonic mucosa predominates. Generally, imaging is performed 48–72 hr after injection of ^{67}Ga citrate. Earlier imaging at 24 or even 6 hr can be performed with good results, although images are better if done later.

Some neoplasms accumulate ^{67}Ga citrate and, as described in Chapter 13, tumor imaging is another important indication for gallium imaging. The precise mechanism of gallium localization in infections remains unclear, but may be related to vascular changes, leukocyte plasma membrane binding, lactoferrin binding at the inflammatory site and/or direct bacterial uptake. It is hypothesized that gallium binds to transferrin receptors on tumor cells. Endocytosis of protein-bound gallium and diffusion across hyperpermeable membranes have also been suggested. Whatever the mechanism, gallium uptake appears to be closely associated with inflammatory cellular reaction.

Since normal abdominal activity poses difficulty in searching for intra-abdominal infection with gallium, ^{111}In leukocyte imaging is preferable. Gallium localizes in infections such as abscesses or phlegmons accompanying pancreatitis or cholecystitis, inflammatory lesions such as peritonitis, even in sterile and in healing wounds. Despite the difficulties, gallium scanning often helps in the search for infection in patients after surgery. Approximately 70–80% of intra-abdominal abscesses are detected.

Gallium accumulates in a variety of pulmonary infections, including pneumococcal pneumonia, anaerobic abscesses, septic emboli, *pneumocystis carinii,* and granulomatous processes such as coccidiomycosis and tuberculosis. Noninfectious gallium-avid pulmonary processes include neoplasm, sarcoidosis, usual interstitial pneumonitis, pneumoconiosis, lupus erythematosus, pulmonary angiogranulomatosis, fibrosing alveolitis, and other active diffuse infiltrative lung diseases.

Although nonspecific, gallium uptake provides a means of sensitive detection of an active pulmonary infection or granulomatous process. Whereas chest roentgenographic findings may not indicate the activity status of an inflammatory process, gallium uptake is very sensitive to inflammatory activity. For example, active tuberculosis typically concentrates gallium, whereas nonactive old tuberculous scars do not. Opportunistic infections in chronically diseased lung take up gallium. Diffuse infiltrative lung diseases in which the chest roentgenogram appears normal may show gallium uptake as well. In these cases, the gallium image can serve as a guide to more aggressive diagnostic procedures, such as biopsy, and as a means for following response to therapy.

Patients with the acquired immunodeficiency syndrome (AIDS) provide an example of the utility of the gallium scan in detecting occult infection as well as monitoring the response to therapy. Because of depression of the cellular immune response due to invasion of the T-lymphocytes with the retrovirus, human immunodeficiency virus (HIV), AIDS victims have a variety of complicating infections including viruses, fungi, protozoa, myco-bacteria and bacteria as well as neoplasms, particularly lympho-ma and Kaposi's sarcoma. The complicating infection is often the presenting complaint of the patient with AIDS. Diffuse pulmon-ary uptake on the gallium scan in the face of a normal chest x-ray occurs with a high enough frequency that the gallium scan has been used to screen for *pneumocystis carinii,* the most common cause of this finding in AIDS patients. More focal abnormalities can occur with bacterial abnormalities and lymph node uptake can be seen with *mycobacterium avium-intracellulare* and *mycobacteri-um tuberculosis* as well as with lymphoma. Conversely, gallium uptake is not present in Kaposi's sarcoma in spite of clear-cut x-ray changes. Gallium imaging can also be used to monitor the response to therapy, as it is a sensitive indicator of the cellular inflammatory response. As the disease responds to therapy, gal-lium uptake diminishes.

Quantitative indices of gallium uptake can be derived if the images are recorded by computer. These data, or semiquan-titative evaluations, are helpful in measuring the response to therapy. Various published reports have documented good cor-relations between the degree and extent of abnormal gallium uptake in the lungs with bronchoalveolar lavage cell counts in many interstitial and alveolar lung inflammatory and granulomatous diseases.

Disc space infections, hematogenous osteomyelitis, or osteomyelitis superimposed on traumatized bone or prosthetic devices are detected on gallium scans. Gallium imaging is highly sensitive in early osteomyelitis (Fig. 12-1) and in detecting re-newed active disease in chronic osteomyelitis. In young children, several reports indicate that the sensitivity and specificity of gal-lium imaging exceed the bone scan. Experimental evidence sug-gests that if gallium is not concentrated in a lesion, active osteomyelitis is extremely unlikely. Caution is warranted, how-

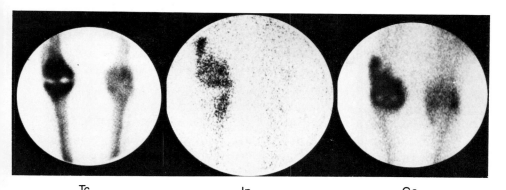

Tc   In   Ga

FIG. 12-1. Technetium-99m MDP bone scan, ^{111}In-labeled leukocyte scan, and ^{67}Ga citrate scan in the same patient with joint space infection and osteomyelitis of the femur and tibia around the right knee. All radiopharmaceuticals show abnormal increased uptake in the involved regions. The indium-labeled leukocyte study shows more extensive involvement of the anteromedial aspect of the tibia than do the gallium and technetium studies. Both the indium and the gallium studies showed collections of abnormal activity in the lateral aspect of the femur, not well seen on the technetium bone scan, perhaps reflecting a soft tissue inflammatory collection in that region.

ever, in the use of gallium in children, since the radiation exposure is considerably higher than that of the ^{99m}Tc bone scan. (See also discussion on osteomyelitis in Chapter 9.)

In cases of fever of unknown origin, gallium is probably the screening imaging procedure of choice, since occult infectious lesions as well as occult tumors can be identified. The whole-body image of the gallium distribution could then serve as a guide for other tests (CT, ultrasound, angiography), if warranted, to characterize an abnormality further.

INDIUM-111-LABELED LEUKOCYTES

Indium-111-labeled autologous leukocyte imaging is also used in detecting infection. Lack of normal accumulation in the abdomen other than in the liver and spleen enhances the sensitivity of indium leukocytes over gallium in detecting intra-abdominal infection. Reports show a high sensitivity exceeding 90% with only a few false-positive studies. False-negative studies are minimized by performing a ^{99m}Tc sulfur colloid liver–spleen scan in conjunction with the ^{111}In-labeled leukocyte images to ensure that no abscesses have been hidden in the normal liver–spleen uptake of indium (Fig. 12-2).

Generally, imaging is performed 24 hr after labeling and reinjecting autologous leukocytes. A 66% decrease in image sensitivity is seen when attempts are made to detect abscesses at 4 hr rather than 24 hr. The labeling process requires care and attention to detail but is easily done within 1½ hr. Indium-111 in the form of oxine or tropolone is used.

Indium-111-labeled leukocytes are also clinically useful in the diagnosis of infection of vascular grafts. There are conflicting reports of the value of this test in identifying bone infection (Fig. 12-1). Comparative experiences with ^{111}In-labeled leukocytes and ^{67}Ga imaging seem to indicate that indium has its highest

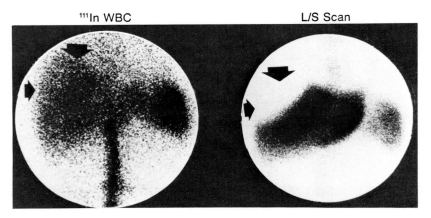

FIG. 12-2. Indium-111 leukocyte anterior scan (*left*) showing the appearance of normal localization in the liver and spleen and linear mid-abdominal uptake corresponding to the incision site in this recently postoperative patient with fever and abdominal pain. Clear identification of a lesion in the upper part of the right lobe of the liver is seen on the accompanying ^{99m}Tc sulfur colloid scan (*right*, lesion is indicated by *arrows*). That region shows ^{111}In leukocyte uptake (*arrows, left*) indicating presence of an abscess. This case emphasizes the importance of correlating the indium images with technetium liver–spleen images.

sensitivity in acute infectious processes, whereas gallium excels in its sensitivity in detecting more chronic infectious lesions. Gallium behaves somewhat as a bone imaging agent with increased uptake at sites of augmented bone osteoblastic activity. Proliferative bone formation at the site of suspected infection that can occur with exuberant callus formation or severe degenerative change will take up gallium, even though no infection is present. In such cases, ^{111}In-labeled leukocytes are preferred over gallium because of the difficulty in interpreting abnormal gallium uptake. Leukocyte uptake is not usually affected by degenerative and traumatic changes in bone, but reliably reflects the migration of leukocytes to the site of infection.

Reported experience in pulmonary lesions indicates that ^{111}In-labeled leukocytes are taken up in a wide variety of pulmonary processes, including pneumonia, empyema, and lung abscesses. Unfortunately, abnormal lung uptake has also been seen in such nonspecific processes as atelectasis, adult respiratory distress syndrome (ARDS), pulmonary embolism, aspiration, and congestive heart failure. Patterns of focal and diffuse uptake have been reported.

SELECTED READINGS

Multiorgan Imaging

Alazraki N. Bone imaging by radionuclide techniques. In: Resnick D, Niwayama A, eds. *Diagnosis of bone and joint disorders.* 2nd ed. Philadelphia: WB Saunders; 1988:460–505

Drum DE. Current status of radiocolloid hepatic scintiphotography for space-occupying disease. *Semin Nucl Med* 1982; 12:64–74

Handmaker H. Nuclear renal imaging in acute pyelonephritis. *Semin Nucl Med* 1982; 12:246–253

Gallium-67 Imaging

Coleman DL, Hattner RS, Luce JM, et al. Correlation between gallium lung scans and fiberoptic bronchoscopy in patients with suspected *Pneumocystis carinii* pneumonia and the acquired immune deficiency syndrome. *Am Rev Resp Dis* 1984; 130:1166–1169

Henkin RE. Gallium-67 in the diagnosis of inflammatory disease. In: Hoffer PB, Beckerman C, Henkin RE, eds. *Gallium-67 imaging.* New York: Wiley, 1978:66–92

Hoffer P. Gallium and infection. *J Nucl Med* 1980; 21:484–488

Lewin JS, Rosenfeld NS, Hoffer PB, et al. Acute osteomyelitis in children: Combined Tc-99m and Ga-67 imaging. *Radiology* 1986; 158:795–804

McNeil BJ, Sanders R, Alderson PO, et al. A prospective study of computed tomography, ultrasound and gallium imaging in patients with fever. *Radiology* 1981; 139:647–653

Staab, EV, McCartney WH. Role of gallium 67 in inflammatory disease. *Semin Nucl Med* 1978; 8:219–234

Indium-111-Labeled Leukocytes

Cook PS, Datz FL, Disbro MA, et al. Clinical significance of pulmonary uptake with indium-111 leukocyte imaging in patients with suspected occult infections. *Radiology* 1984; 150:557–561

Knochel JQ, Koehler PR, Lee TG, et al. Diagnosis of abdominal abscesses with computed tomography, ultrasound and 111 In leukocyte scans. *Radiology* 1980; 137:425–432

McDougall IR, Baumert JE, Lantieri RL. Evaluation of 111 In leukocyte whole body scanning. *AJR* 1979; 133:849–854

Propst–Proctor SL, Dillingham MF, McDougall IR, Goodwin D. The white blood cell scan in orthopedics. *Clin Orthop* 1982; 168:157–165

Thakur ML, Lavender JP, Arnot RN, et al. Indium-111-labeled autologous leukocytes in man. *J Nucl Med* 1977; 18:1014–1019

13
Cancer

The sensitivity and specificity of available radionuclide imaging methods in detecting primary neoplasms and their metastases varies with tumor type and location. For some processes, radionuclide imaging may provide the best available means of documenting the presence or absence of disease, as in spread of functioning differentiated thyroid cancer. For some primary tumors such as pancreatic cancer, ultrasound and computed tomography (CT) imaging are far more helpful. Rapid development of ultrasound and CT and the addition of digital angiography and magnetic resonance imaging (MRI) to conventional radiologic techniques offer a plethora of possibilities for evaluating the cancer patient. Algorithms for workup must be individualized to the tumor type and vary according to institutional resources. This section focuses on nuclear medicine techniques used to evaluate neoplasms in different body regions. It also illustrates the role of nuclear medicine in four common malignancies: non-oat cell lung carcinoma and adenocarcinoma of the breast, colon, and prostate. The reader is also referred to the chapters that deal with specific organs affected by cancer (see Chapters 3 and 6–10).

RADIONUCLIDE LIVER IMAGING

Radionuclide hepatic imaging is a cost-effective, sensitive method for detecting hepatic metastases when there is hepatomegaly or elevation of liver enzymes, or both. On the basis of a tumor doubling time of ~1–4 mo, and the approximate limit of a 1.5-cm diameter for visualization of an intrahepatic mass (see earlier discussion on liver scintigraphy, Chapter 6), a metastatic focus may well have been present for several years before it can be detected by radionuclide imaging. True-positive results are found in 75–90% of patients with pathologically proved liver lesions. Recent studies report that sensitivity of SPECT imaging for detecting hepatic lesions is 5–10% superior to radionuclide planar imaging. Before they grow large enough to be resolved as discrete defects, hepatic metastases may appear as uneven activity on the radionuclide image. The finding of multiple defects on the liver scan is not specific for metastatic disease. When warranted, other imaging modalities are also employed. For example, the gallium scan can identify infection or tumor (see Fig. 13-1); ultrasound can distinguish between cystic and solid processes; and CT scanning with contrast enhancement can confirm the presence or absence of a lesion and add density information to contribute to the differential diagnosis. Considerations of cost,

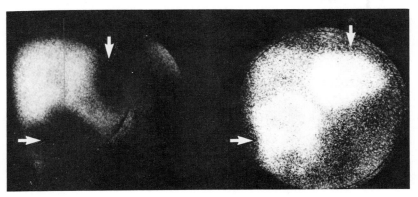

$^{99m}Tc_2S_7$ Scan ^{67}Ga Citrate Scan

FIG. 13-1. (*Left*) Anterior view of liver scan using ^{99m}Tc sulfur colloid shows two large foci (*arrows*) representing lesions. The radiocolloid liver scan is nonspecific; these lesions could be tumors, abscesses, hematomas, cysts, or other benign lesions. (*Right*) Anterior view of the liver gallium scan shows that these regions concentrate gallium (*arrows*) indicating that they represent either tumor or infection. The patient has primary adenocarcinoma of the colon and metastases to the liver.

sensitivity, lack of morbidity, and an imaging characterization of hepatic function give radionuclide liver imaging a prominent role in screening for liver metastases.

RADIONUCLIDE LYMPHOSCINTIGRAPHY

Radionuclide lymphoscintigraphy is a safe reproducible, easily performed, and well-tolerated examination that uses radiocolloids to image regional lymph channels and lymph nodes. The technique offers the opportunity for repetitive studies in following patients with nodal metastases or for assessing the effects of surgical therapies in benign conditions, such as lymphedema. Advantages over other radiologic techniques for visualizing lymph nodes and lymph channels include (1) a more physiologic assessment of lymph flow, since the injected material is in a volume of 0.1–0.2 ml; (2) an easy rapid injection technique which requires no skin incision; (3) an ability to visualize normal size (1–4 mm) nodes; and (4) the capacity to define early micrometastatic lymph node involvement.

Lymphatic groups about which a reasonable body of information using this technique has been gathered include the internal mammary nodes, lymphatics of the trunk and extremities and lymph nodes of the iliopelvic group. The preferred radiocolloid for this study is ^{99m}Tc antimony trisulfide colloid, a small particle 0.001–0.01 μm in size.

Internal Mammary Lymphoscintigraphy

One of the most widely used lymphoscintigraphic techniques is visualization of the internal mammary nodes in breast cancer patients undergoing radiation therapy planning or being evaluated for occult metastatic involvement of these nodes. Three hours following transdermal injection into the posterior rectus sheath in the subcostal area, lymph channels are routinely visualized and may be evaluated for drainage patterns and symmetry of filling (Fig. 13-2). Not only may lymphatic abnormalities be detected, but abnormal nodes that should be included in the

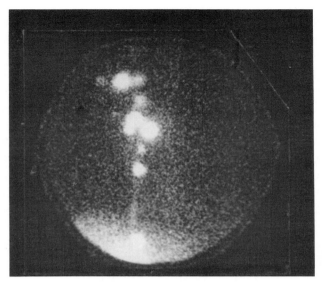

FIG. 13-2. Anterior view of the thorax obtained 3 hr following a right subcostal injection of antimony trisulfide colloid reveals the right internal mammary lymph channel and multiple lymph nodes between the xyphoid and supraclavicular region. Diffuse uptake at the lower edge of the image represents radiocolloid that passed through the lymphatic channel into the general circulation, to be sequestered by the liver.

radiation treatment field are localized, leading to a more rational, individualized therapeutic approach for breast carcinoma.

Intradermal Lymphoscintigraphy

A more superficial intradermal injection allows visualization of cutaneous lymphatic pathways and has direct application for staging truncal melanomas and evaluating congenital or acquired extremity lymphedema.

For defining lymphatic drainage from malignant melanoma presenting on the trunk, results from this pre- or perioperative procedure provide critical data for planning "curative" surgery. There are frequent exceptions to the classically described anatomic lymphatic drainage pathways in this disease and, before performing major ablative surgery, the full extent of potential dissemination can be defined by radionuclide scintigraphy. The appearance of lymphatic groups distant from the expected principal drainage site of the primary lesion occurs in more than one-half of patients studied and has obvious impact on the type and extent of surgery.

Intradermal injection of radiocolloid in the dorsum of the hands or feet has been used to define pre- and postoperative lymphatic anatomy and function in patients with lymphedema. Imaging is performed immediately and for up to 3 hr or more after injection. With respect to image interpretation, results do not differentiate between primary and secondary lymphedema; the scintigraphic patterns do not correlate with the duration of symptoms; it may be necessary to have the patient elevate the affected extremity for 1–2 days prior to the study in an effort toward optimal visualization of any surgically available lymph channels.

Iliopelvic Lymphoscintigraphy

Injections made deep into the ischiorectal fossa allow visualization of the internal and common iliac lymph nodes, which are those at risk of involvement in common genitourinary malignancies. Three hours postinjection, an elegant depiction of these deep lymphatic structures can be scintigraphically recorded and conclusions drawn as to the presence of nodal metastases.

EVALUATION OF THE CHEST

Lung

The plain chest roentgenogram offers a simple, harmless means of evaluating the lung for parenchymal nodules, the bones for pathologic anatomic changes, and the hila and mediastinum for masses. Although it remains the traditional time-honored screening procedure, the plain x-ray film provides neither sensitive nor specific information. Radionuclide perfusion lung images may define disproportionate perfusion deficits attributable to bronchogenic carcinoma, unexpected from an x-ray film of the chest. These findings are clinically useful in patients being considered for surgery who have severely compromised pulmonary function. Quantitation of regional function may provide information critical for the decision to perform a lung resection.

Radionuclide scanning of the chest with iodide for functioning differentiated thyroid cancer metastases and ^{99m}Tc diphosphonate bone imaging for parenchymal lung metastases from osteogenic sarcoma are examples of techniques showing relatively high specificity.

Bony Thorax

Bone scintigraphy of the thorax, as part of a whole-body scan, localizes increased bone turnover and hence metastases, more sensitively than does bone radiography. The bone scan is the imaging modality of choice for staging prostate cancer. The value of the bone scan in screening asymptomatic patients with clinically early breast and lung cancer has been debated, but there is no doubt that this technique will detect bone metastases that are not otherwise clinically apparent.

Mediastinum

Gallium scintigraphy of the thorax for localization of primary bronchogenic carcinoma and for detecting mediastinal involvement provides a means of determining tumor resectability. Unfortunately, as with most radionuclide studies, gallium uptake is not specific for neoplasm and is also seen in other pathologic processes, including infections and inflammatory lesions. The sensitivity of gallium in detecting lung cancer is ~80–85%. Gallium is also used in detecting the extent of lymphoma in the chest with a reported sensitivity of ~75–80%.

Studies have found that when the primary lung cancer concentrated gallium, imaging of the mediastinum for abnormal gallium uptake as an indicator of metastases showed a sensitivity of 81–100% for the gallium mediastinal scan, as compared with mediastinoscopies. The criteria for what constitutes positive mediastinal uptake varies, accounting for some of the reported discrepancies. The true specificity (i.e., the ratio of the number of true-negative gallium mediastinum scans to the number of negative mediastinoscopies) varied between 53 and 86%.

Studies to define the best nonsurgical modality for staging lung cancer are ongoing in many institutions, comparing gallium (Fig. 13-3), SPECT imaging, and CT mediastinal scans. The CT scan is remarkably sensitive in detecting mediastinal tumor nodes as small as 1 cm and is not limited by tumor type as is gallium, which does not concentrate in adenocarcinomas as well as in some other types of tumors. However, gallium may detect mediastinal involvement if there is high level uptake in metastases that may not be apparent on the CT image because of size

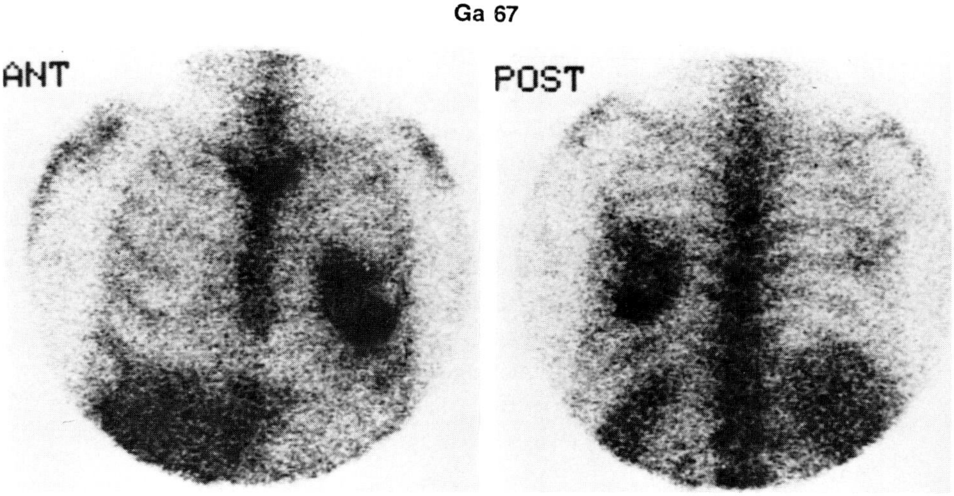

Ga 67

FIG. 13-3. Gallium-67 citrate images in anterior and posterior views in a patient with bronchogenic carcinoma. The images show uptake of gallium in the primary lung cancer located in the left mid-lung field. There is clear separation of the abnormal tumor uptake from the mediastinal region indicating no mediastinal spread of the tumor. This finding was confirmed at thoracotomy.

or location. SPECT imaging is currently being evaluated, but appears to be promising for improving the sensitivity of gallium mediastinal scans for detection of lung cancer metastases.

Heart

Radionuclide methods for calculating left ventricular ejection fraction are a sensitive means of monitoring cardiotoxic effects of chemotherapeutic agents, such as Adriamycin. Such data permit individualization of dose regimens. A decreasing ejection fraction may be seen well before any clinical effects become apparent and permits appropriate adjustment of Adriamycin dose before irreversible damage occurs.

RADIOIMMUNODETECTION AND RADIOIMMUNOTHERAPY

The potential of radionuclides for detecting and treating cancer has been recognized for decades. Most tumor-seeking tracers, such as ^{67}Ga citrate, are not specific for neoplasms and show varying degrees of normal or inflammatory tissue activity. A major challenge has been to target the radionuclide exclusively to neoplastic tissue. In theory, it might be possible to exploit physiology unique to neoplasms to deliver the radionuclides selectively to neoplastic tissue, but in practice this has been possible with only a few types of cancer, such as thyroid carcinoma, which can be effectively treated with ^{131}I. Monoclonal antibodies labeled with appropriate radionuclides provide the potential for specific delivery of radionuclides to a particular cancer for detection and treatment. In this section, tumor refers to malignant neoplasm.

The first radiolabeled antitumor antibodies were prepared from the serum of animals inoculated with neoplastic cells, cell extracts or cellular antigens, such as carcinoembryonic antigen (CEA). These heterosera contained polyclonal antibodies, that is, mixtures of antibodies having varying specificities for the tumor and for other tissue. Radiolabeled polyclonal antibodies were used in diagnostic imaging to localize tumor tissue, but the images generally had considerable activity in other tissues, particularly in the blood. By contrast, monoclonal antibodies produced using hybridoma technology are directed against relatively specific antigenic determinants of the neoplastic cell; the more specific the antigen is for tumor cells, the less activity the labeled monoclonal antibody against that antigen will show in normal tissues. Since some epitopes on tumor cells may be shared by normal tissues, current investigations are directed at producing monoclonal antibodies or antibody fragments that have minimal cross-reactivity with normal tissues.

Radiolabeled monoclonal antibodies are currently being evaluated for imaging a number of different tumors. Preliminary results in cancers with well-characterized antibodies to relatively specific antigens, such as in melanoma and cutaneous T-cell lymphoma, have been very encouraging. The latter is unique in that the antigen–antibody reaction may take place on the surface of circulating neoplastic cells, which are then sequestered in lymph nodes. An example of ^{111}In-labeled antibody imaging is shown in Fig. 13-4.

Most hybridomas used to produce monoclonal antibodies have been of murine origin. When antibodies of mouse origin are administered to human beings, they are recognized as foreign protein and induce formation of human antimurine antibodies. Antibody fragments are somewhat less immunogenic than whole antibody and clear more rapidly from the blood although they may have greater localization in the liver. Successive administration, even of antibody fragments, will induce antibodies that prevent their localization in tumor precluding further diagnostic or therapeutic applications. Alternative methods of monoclonal antibody production may avoid the problem of inducing human antimurine antibody formation; such methods include production of human/mouse antibodies using recombinant DNA techniques, as well as formation of hybridomas from human cell lines.

Preliminary studies of cancer therapy with radiolabeled monoclonal antibodies as well as some polyclonal antibodies have been promising. Radionuclide labels such as ^{123}I, ^{99m}Tc, and

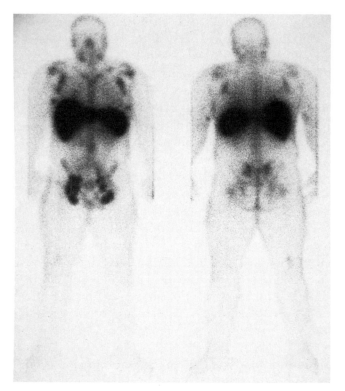

FIG. 13-4. Anterior and posterior whole-body images using ^{111}In-labeled T 101 monoclonal antibody in a patient with cutaneous T-cell lymphoma. Prominent labeled antibody activity is evident in tumor containing axillary and inguinal lymph nodes as well as in tumor cells in the skin. Activity is also present normally in the liver, spleen and bone marrow. (Reproduced with permission of the author and Pergamon Press from Larson et al., *Nucl Med Biol* 1986; 13:207.)

[111]In have desirable imaging properties and, because of short half-lives, deliver low radiation doses; however for the same reason, they are unsuitable for therapy, which requires high radiation doses. An ideal label for therapy should remain on the antibody until it reaches the cancer, reside in the tumor tissue through several half-lives, and deliver a high radiation dose to the cancer. Possible radionuclides for therapy include ^{131}I, other β-particle emitters, and α-particle emitters.

SPECIFIC TUMOR TYPES

Adenocarcinoma of the Breast

Skeletal metastases occur in ~40% of patients with breast cancer who are found to have metastases. Clinically overt metastatic spread of breast cancer to local nodes, subcutaneous tissue, lungs, or bones can be documented in 75–90% of such patients by physical examination, x-ray film of the chest, and bone scan. Abnormal bone scans are found in 2% of patients designated as having Stage I disease on the basis of pathologic findings and in 7% of those classified as Stage II.

Other causes of abnormal bone scans besides metastases, include recent or old trauma, benign neoplasm, and degenerative changes, so that the true positive yield in screening all patients undergoing axillary dissection may not be sufficiently high to predict which patient has metastatic disease. By selecting from patients who underwent biopsy and axillary sampling before definitive therapy, those with four or more histologically involved nodes or high axillary node involvement or both, bone-scanning predictivity would be improved. Approximately 20–25% of patients with Stage III disease have abnormal bone scans. This discovery before radical surgical therapy may help institute a more rational therapeutic approach.

Visualization of the presence or absence of involvement of the internal mammary lymph nodes and their location permits rational individualization of radiation therapy (see discussion under internal mammary scintigraphy, p. 159). Figure 13-2 shows a normal configuration and drainage pattern of right internal mammary lymph nodes in a patient with breast carcinoma.

Non-Oat Cell Bronchogenic Carcinoma

Bronchogenic cancer spreads via the lymphatic drainage system to local, hilar, carinal, and mediastinal nodes. Mediastinal or chest wall involvement precludes surgical cure, and such patients are usually irradiated. Approximately one-third of patients thought to have resectable cancers on the basis of physical examination, chest film, and bronchoscopy will be proved to have a nonresectable lesion, usually by mediastinoscopy.

Gallium scintigraphy detects 83–90% of histologically proved squamous cell carcinomas and 75% of adenocarcinomas, although size is a major factor, since only 43% of lesions < 2 cm are detectable. The ability of gallium imaging to demonstrate a pulmonary parenchymal neoplasm (85%) exceeds its ability to demonstrate regional node involvement (72%) or distant metastases (60%). Liver metastases occur in 40–44% of patients with bronchogenic carcinomas, so that radionuclide liver imaging is useful. Skeletal metastases are also common, occurring in 31–40% of cases, as are brain metastases (28–44%). Liver, bone, and brain scans are generally not performed routinely, but are reserved for patients who show symptoms indicating disease in those organs. Few patients with a positive bone or liver scan have long to live, and most die from their disease within 1 year.

Adenocarcinoma of the Bowel

Many patients with adenocarcinoma of the large bowel have distant metastatic disease when they first seek medical attention. One-half of these patients die because of problems related to recurrence of local disease. Distant metastases most frequently involve the liver (65%) (see Fig. 6-3, p. 86) and lungs (28%). The value of the liver scan and x-ray film of the chest is apparent. Bone scanning is warranted only in symptomatic patients, as skeletal metastases occur in fewer than 10% of patients with primary colon cancer. Screening by brain scan or head CT should be reserved for those patients displaying clinical signs or symptoms of intracerebral disease.

Prostate Cancer

Prostatic cancer metastasizes most commonly to bone (see Figs. 9-1, p. 115, and 13-5). At the time of initial staging, various

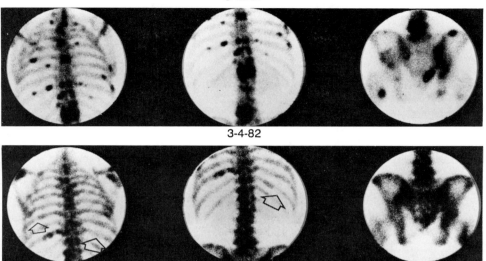

FIG. 13-5. Technetium-99m MDP bone scans in a patient with widespread metastatic prostate cancer to the bones. (**Top**) Multiple focal regions of increased uptake consistent with bony metastases in the ribs, the spine, and the pelvis. (**Bottom**) Approximately 6.5 mo later, the images show even more widespread dissemination of metastases in the bones (easily misinterpreted by a novice as showing more normal appearing bones). In fact, nearly every bone imaged is infiltrated with tumor, so that individual lesions do not stand out as more abnormal than adjacent bone. Some cold foci, probably representing more complete replacement of bone by tumor, involving ribs are evident (*arrows*).

reported series indicate true-positive metastatic bone lesions on bone scans in 30–46% of patients. At autopsy, 50–70% of patients with prostate cancer are found to have bone metastases. When the patient first seeks medical attention, the relative sensitivities of other diagnostic modalities, assuming a relative value of 1.00 for bone scanning, are approximately as follows: skeletal survey, 0.68; alkaline phosphatase, 0.54–0.77; and acid phosphatase, as determined by standard enzyme assays, 0.5–0.6. Liver scanning should be reserved for patients with hepatomegaly or abnormal elevation of hepatic enzymes in the serum.

SELECTED READINGS

Radionuclide Liver Imaging

Alderson PO, Adams DF, McNeil BJ, et al. Computed tomography, ultrasound, and scintigraphy of the liver in patients with colon or breast carcinoma: A prospective comparison. *Radiology* 1983; 149:225–230

Drum DE, Beard JM. Scintigraphic criteria for hepatic metastases from cancer of the colon and breast. *J Nucl Med* 1976; 13:677–680

Harbert JC: Efficacy of bone and liver scanning in malignant diseases: Facts and opinions. In: Freeman LM, Weissmann HS, eds. *Nuclear medicine annual 1982*. New York: Raven Press; 1982:373–401

Lunia S, Parthasarthy KL, Bakshi S, et al. An evaluation of 99m Tc sulfur colloid liver scintiscans and their usefulness in metastatic workup—A review of 1424 studies. *J Nucl Med* 1975; 16: 62–65

Patton DD. Current status of liver scintigraphy for space occupying disease. In: Freeman LM, Weissmann HS, eds. *Nuclear medicine annual 1982*. New York: Raven Press; 1982:35–79

Petasnik JP, Ram P, Turner DA, et al. The relationship of computed tomography, gray scale ultrasonography and radionuclide imaging in the evaluation of hepatic masses. *Semin Nucl Med* 1981; 11:8–21

Lung

Alazraki N. Usefulness of gallium imaging in the evaluation of lung cancer. *CRC Crit Rev Diagn Imag* 1980; 13(3):249–267

DeLand FH, Sauerbrunn BJL, Boyd C, et al. [67]Gallium-citrate imaging in untreated primary lung cancer: Preliminary report of cooperative group. *J Nucl Med* 1974; 15:408–411

Gravenstein S, Peltz MA, Pories W. How ominous is an abnormal scan in bronchogenic carcinoma? *JAMA* 1979; 241:2523–2524

Kelly RJ, Cowan RJ, Ferree CB, et al. Efficacy of radionuclide scanning in patients with lung cancer. *JAMA* 1979; 242:2855–2857

Koh HK, Prout MN. The efficient workup of suspected lung cancer. *Arch Intern Med* 1982; 142:966–968

Lymphoscintigraphy

Ege GN. Lymphoscintigraphy—Techniques and applications in the management of breast carcinoma. *Semin Nucl Med* 1983; 13: 26–34

Mediastinum

Alazraki NP, Ramsdell JW, Taylor A, et al. Reliability of the gallium scan chest radiography compared to mediastinoscopy for evaluating mediastinal spread in lung cancer. *Am Rev Respir Dis* 1978; 117:415–420

DeMeester FR, Golomb HM, Kirchner P, et al. The role of gallium 67 scanning in the clinical staging and preoperative evaluation of patients with carcinoma of the lung. *Ann Thorac Surg* 1979; 28:451–464

Radioimmunodetection, Radioimmunotherapy

Carrasquillo JA, Bunn PA, Keenan AM, et al. Radioimmunodetection of cutaneous T-cell lymphoma with ^{111}In-labeled T101 monoclonal antibody. *N Engl J Med* 1986; 315:673–680

DeNardo GL, DeNardo SJ. Perspectives on the future of radioimmunodiagnosis and radioimmunotherapy of cancer. In: Burchiel SW, Rhodes BA, eds. *Radioimmunoimaging and radioimmunotherapy*. New York: Elsevier; 1983:41–62

Grossman ZD, Rosebrough SF. *Clinical radioimmunoimaging*. New York: Grune & Stratton; 1988

Halpern SE, Stern P, Hagan PL, et al. The labeling of monoclonal antibodies with indium-111: Technique and advantages compared to radioiodine labeling. In: Burchiel SW, Rhodes BA, eds. *Radioimmunoimaging and radioimmunotherapy*. New York: Elsevier; 1983:197–206

Larson SM, Brown JP, Wright PW, et al. Imaging of melanoma with I-131-labeled monoclonal antibodies. *J Nucl Med* 1983; 24:123–129

Larson SM, Carrasquillo JA, Reynolds, JC, et al. Therapeutic applications of radiolabeled antibodies: Current situation and prospects. *Nucl Med Biol* 1986; 13:207–213

Moldofsky PJ, Sears HF, Mulhern CB Jr, et al. Detection of metastatic tumor in normal-sized retroperitoneal lymph nodes by monoclonal antibody imaging. *N Engl J Med* 1984; 311:106–107

Sun LK, Curtis P, Rakowicz-Szulczynska E, et al. Chimeric antibody with human constant regions and mouse variable regions directed against carcinoma-associated antigen 17-1A. *Proc Natl Acad Sci USA* 1987; 84:214–218

Breast

Gerber PH, Goodreau JJ, Kirchner PT, et al. Efficacy of preoperative and postoperative bone scanning in management of breast carcinoma. *N Engl J Med* 1977; 297:300–303

McNeil BJ. Rationale for the use of bone scans in selected metastatic and primary bone tumors. *Semin Nucl Med* 1978; 8:336–345

Pistenma DA, McDougall IR, Kriss JP. Screening for bone metastases. Are only scans necessary? *JAMA* 1980; 231:46–50

Prostate

Jacobs SC. Spread of prostate cancer to bone. *Urology* 1982; 21:337–344

McNeil BJ, Polak JF. An update on the rationale for the use of bone scans in selected metastatic and primary bone tumors. In: Pauwels EK, Schutte HE, Taconis WK, eds. *Bone scintigraphy.* The Hague: Leiden University Press; 1981

Shafer RB, Reinke DB. Contribution of the bone scan, serum acid and alkaline phosphatase, and the radiographic bone survey to the management of newly diagnosed carcinoma of the prostate. *Clin Nucl Med* 1977; 6:200–203

Nonimaging Diagnostic Techniques

14

Nonimaging Procedures

Nonimaging nuclear medicine encompasses two types of procedures: (1) radioimmunoassay (RIA) to quantitate biologically important substances in the serum or other body fluids (in vitro procedures), and (2) evaluation of physiologic function by administering small tracer amounts of radioactive materials to patients, and then subsequently counting specimens of urine, blood, feces, or breath. A wide variety of physiologic phenomena may be measured, including vitamin B_{12} absorption (Schilling test), fat absorption, ability to deconjugate bile acids, red cell survival and sequestration, red cell mass, plasma volume, various body space measurements, ferrokinetics, and total body water. In contrast to RIA, these procedures require the administration of small amounts of radioactivity to the patient, usually yielding radiation exposures less than that given by a conventional x-ray film of the chest.

RADIOLIGAND ASSAYS

Berson and Yalow developed, and in 1960 described, radioimmunoassay (RIA) work for which Yalow received the Nobel Price for Medicine in 1977. The usefulness of RIA stems from its high sensitivity, detecting a variety of hormones and drugs in concentrations as low as 10^{-12} moles/liter or less. In addition to its high sensitivity, RIA is also extremely specific because of the inherent specificity of the antibody produced against the antigen

175

to be measured. Not all in vitro radioassays involve antibody, and other binding agents (ligands) may be used. As an example of the specificity of the antigen–antibody reaction, thyroxine (T_4) can be differentiated from triiodothyronine (T_3), even though these molecules differ by only one iodide atom.

Competitive ligand binding is the basis of RIA, generally called radioligand assay. A typical RIA uses a limited quantity of antibody, usually immunoglobulin G (IgG) specific for the antigen to be measured, radiolabeled antigen, known unlabeled standards of known antigen concentration, and the unknown sample containing the same antigen that is to be measured. A series of test tubes containing identical concentrations of radiolabeled antigen as well as a fixed amount of antibody is prepared. Either the known standard antigen preparations, or the unknown sample, are added to these tubes. Incubation permits an antigen–antibody reaction to occur:

$$\text{Antigen + radiolabeled antigen + antibody (limited)}$$
$$\downarrow \quad \uparrow$$
Antigen–antibody complex + radiolabeled antigen–
antibody complex + surplus (free) antigen
+ surplus (free) radiolabeled antigen

Increasing antigen concentration decreases the percentage of radiolabeled antigen bound to the limited quantity of antibody. The added antigen competes for limited antibody binding sites. Antigen bound to antibody is then separated from free antigen by means of one or a combination of several techniques. Free antigen may be adsorbed on charcoal; the antigen–antibody complex can be precipitated with salt, solvents, or a second antibody; or, the antigen–antibody reaction can occur on a solid surface, such as a test tube wall or a particle. Radioactivity in the two antigen fractions, bound or free, may be measured in the gamma counter.

A standard curve is then drawn, plotting the bound: free radioactivity ratio on the ordinate against the known standard concentration of the antigen measured on the abscissa. By comparing the bound:free ratio of the unknown sample with the standard curve, antigen concentration in the unknown sample is determined.

Clinical Uses of RIA

RIA is currently used to detect and measure a wide variety of biologically important substances. Serum hormone levels, for example, are principally measured by this technique.

Thyroid hormone studies are among the most commonly performed RIA procedures. In serum, T_4 and T_3 circulate bound to thyroid-binding proteins, principally thyroxine-binding globulin (TBG). The binding affinity of TBG for T_3 is much less than that for T_4. This weaker binding, in conjunction with its higher affinity for cellular receptors, accounts for the greater mole-for-mole metabolic potency of T_3 compared with T_4. Metabolic activity correlates best with a small serum fraction of unbound thyroid hormone called free T_4 (0.05%) and free T_3 (0.5%). However, measurement of total T_4 or T_3 proves much more practical, in that it is faster and less costly. Measurement of the total T_4 or T_3 presents an accurate reflection of the active free fraction of each, and hence, thyroid hormone production, provided the TBG concentration is within normal limits.

If the TBG capacity is increased, the total T_4 and T_3 levels may be elevated in the face of normal free hormone levels (i.e., in euthyroid patients). Clinical conditions that can elevate TBG include pregnancy, estrogen administration (e.g., oral contraceptives), liver disease, and TBG levels during the first few weeks of life. Conversely, if the TBG level is depressed, such as in the nephrotic syndrome, chronic illness, or androgen administration, a low T_4 level may be found in a euthyroid patient.

In order to determine the amount of TBG capacity, a so-called serum resin T_3 uptake test can be performed. This test is an index of unoccupied TBG sites for either T_3 or T_4 and is not a measure of circulating T_3. By comparing the T_3 resin uptake with total T_4, an index of free T_4 can be calculated. The chemical equilibrium equation may be written as follows:

Free T_4 + unsaturated TBG sites $\rightleftarrows$ T_4 bound to TBG

Written as a mass action equilibrium reaction and solving for the concentration of free T_4 $[T_4]$:

$$[T_4] = \frac{[T_4 \bullet TBG]}{[TBG] \times K}$$

or is proportional to

$$\frac{[T_4 \bullet TBG]}{[TBG]} = \text{free } T_4 \text{ index},$$

where K is an equilibrium constant and total T_4 approximates $[T_4 \bullet TBG]$ and the T_3 resin uptake is proportional to $[TBG]$. The more laborious dialysis method of measuring free T_4 is rarely used clinically.

Although thyroid studies using radioactivity and the immunoassay technique are those most frequently performed—T_4, T_3, T_3 resin uptake, and thyroid-stimulating hormone (TSH)—many other hormones and drugs such as digoxin and antibiotic levels are routinely assayed by RIA (see the Appendix). These assays serve as the data backbone of many branches of clinical medicine and also make possible investigations creating new medical frontiers.

SCHILLING TEST

Insidious in onset, often vague in symptom presentation, vitamin B_{12} deficiency requires early diagnosis to prevent debilitating anemia, spinal cord degeneration, and death. Although the serum B_{12} level can readily be measured by radioligand assay, the causes of vitamin B_{12} deficiency are not obvious from this assay alone and may include the following:

I. Inadequate intake (rare)
II. Malabsorption

A. Gastric abnormalities
  1. Absence of intrinsic factor (pernicious anemia), gastrectomy
  2. Excess HCl (Zollinger-Ellison syndrome)
B. Intestinal malabsorption
  1. Destruction, removal, or invasion of ileal absorption sites
  2. Competition for B_{12} (fish tapeworm, bacterial overgrowth in small bowel lesions)
  3. Pancreatic disease
  4. Drugs (p-aminosalicylic acid, neomycin, colchicine, calcium-chelating agents)
C. Genetic abnormality in transport proteins

Serum levels of vitamin B_{12} can be measured directly by a radioimmunoassay. In the clinical setting, however, a normal serum vitamin B_{12} result may not exclude a problem in vitamin B_{12} absorption. Administration of vitamin B_{12} by injection is common and serum levels may be temporarily normal for many weeks.

The Schilling test differentiates pernicious anemia from the other listed causes of vitamin B_{12} malabsorption and can establish the functional absence of intrinsic factor when serum B_{12} deficiency or anemia is not yet present or when the patient has received folate or vitamin B_{12} therapy. In the first stage Schilling test, sometime within 1–2 hr following oral administration of cobalt-57-labeled vitamin B_{12}, a flushing dose of 1 mg of nonradioactive vitamin B_{12} is administered subcutaneously or intramuscularly. This procedure ensures that any radioactive vitamin B_{12} absorbed into the blood from the gut finds normal binding sites (principally in the liver) saturated and will be excreted in the urine sample, which is collected over a 24-hr period. The collection period can be extended in renal failure.

The amount of radioactive vitamin B_{12} in the urine is counted. If the amount is low, the study is repeated, this time administering intrinsic factor orally along with the radiolabeled vitamin B_{12} (the Stage II Schilling test). If the low absorption and excretion of the radiolabeled vitamin B_{12} was due to lack of intrinsic factor, absorption will return to normal with the supplied intrinsic factor although rare individuals will not respond to the routinely administered hog intrinsic factor, but will respond to bovine intrinsic factor. If intrinsic factor fails to correct the vitamin B_{12} malabsorption, the cause of malabsorption is established as being due to an abnormality other than intrinsic factor deficit.

Simultaneous administration of cobalt-58- (^{58}Co) labeled vitamin B_{12} and ^{57}Co-labeled vitamin B_{12} complexed with intrinsic factor has been used to perform both the Stage I and Stage II Schilling tests at the same time using a single urine specimen, since their different energy levels enable the separate counting of ^{57}Co and ^{58}Co and permit the conclusion of the test in one day. While some have found this to be a more accurate means of establishing the presence or absence of intrinsic factor deficit, some isotopic exchange apparently takes place and potentially invalidates this approach. This has led to removal of this dual reagent from commercial production.

In the case of bacterial overgrowth (B.2 in the above outline), administration of oral antibiotics corrects the absorption defect on repeat study; similarly, exogenous pancreatic enzyme administration does so in pancreatic insufficiency (indicated as B.3 in the above outline). Lack of pancreatic enzyme impairs the binding to available intrinsic factor, since pancreatic enzyme is required to cleave vitamin B_{12} from nonspecific binding to gastric protein before it can bind to intrinsic factor to form the complex which is required for absorption. Supplying the enzyme corrects this problem. In intestinal malabsorption, none of these additions corrects the malabsorption of radiolabeled vitamin B_{12}.

MEASURING BODY SPACES

The isotope dilution principle can be employed with a variety of selected labeled tracers to measure the spaces in which they are distributed. The principle is based on the fact that the amount of tracer put into a space equals the counts-per-unit volume of the space in which it is distributed times the volume:

$$Q = CV,$$

where Q is the quantity (total counts) of labeled material injected, C is the concentration (counts-per-unit volume) of the labeled tracer sampled after equilibrium has taken place, and V is the volume in which the tracer is distributed. Q, the amount of tracer put into the volume, may be obtained by measuring a standard of the tracer (a duplicate of the sample used), or by measuring the entire injectate before administration. C may be determined by obtaining a sample from the space to be measured and counting the activity in a unit volume (e.g., a milliliter of plasma or whole blood). From these measurements, the volume can be calculated. The validity of this approach assumes that all the tracer material has been injected into the space to be measured, the tracer is uniformly distributed in the space to be measured, the tracer remains only in the space to be measured and does not leak out, and the sample obtained accurately represents the tracer concentration throughout the volume. Such assumptions are rarely completely fulfilled in clinical practice, but careful tracer selection and attention to appropriate equilibrium requirements provide accuracy sufficient for clinical purposes. A common clinical use of this principle is the measurement of blood volume.

Blood Volume

Determination of total blood volume, plasma volume, and red cell mass may be useful in the diagnosis and management of pathophysiologic disorders such as polycythemia rubra vera. Blood volume is defined as the sum of plasma volume and circulating erythrocyte volume. The volume of circulating erythrocytes is constant in normally hydrated human beings and varies little from day to day. Uniform mixing of isotopically labeled erythrocytes within the vascular space is complete within ~20 min after injection, except in cases of shock or severe dehydration. In contrast, the plasma volume is not as constant and fluctuates considerably, depending on the state of hydration.

Loss of a significant quantity of blood over a short period of time might not be reflected immediately in a decreased hematocrit; knowledge of plasma volume then becomes important. The hematocrit, which is an expression of the fractional volume of erythrocytes in a blood sample, varies within the vascular tree as a function of the caliber of the blood vessels through which the blood is flowing. The whole-body hematocrit is an expression of the ratio of erythrocyte volume to total blood volume. Although it is difficult to determine a single numerical figure that relates the peripheral hematocrit to the whole-body hematocrit in various disease states, it is known that in healthy steady-state persons this ratio is ~0.92.

The principle of isotope dilution is employed in nuclear medicine to determine the plasma volume and the erythrocyte volume independently, with the sum of these being equal to the total blood volume. In clinical practice, plasma volume is measured by intravenous injection of ^{125}I-labeled human serum albumin simultaneously with chromium-51- (^{51}Cr) labeled autologous red blood cells. The albumin is distributed in the plasma volume and the cells in the cellular portion of whole blood. Whereas the labeled albumin can be purchased commercially, the red cells must be labeled individually for each patient by taking a sample of the patient's blood, mixing it with ^{51}Cr sodium chromate, and allowing 15 or 20 min to elapse for cell labeling. Both the plasma volume and the red cell volume may be determined from blood samples drawn 10, 20, and 30 min after injection.

Although reports have appeared in the literature suggesting that the plasma volume or the red cell volume can be calculated accurately by simply measuring the former or the latter, this approach does not take into account the variation of peripheral to central and overall hematocrit, and the inaccuracies in measuring the hematocrit. Dependence on measured hematocrit to derive a total blood volume from a calculated plasma volume, for example, substantially increases the error in calculated blood volume.

In addition to the inherent errors in methodology of measuring blood volume, absolute normal values vary with body habitus and are difficult to predict for a given patient. Nonetheless, the test may be helpful in clinical patient management, for diagnosis, and for following changes in volumes in response to therapy.

In some clinical situations such as hypovolemic shock, necessitating accurate calculation of blood volume, conditions for tracer equilibrium and uniform tracer distribution are not met, particularly in the case of albumin, which may extravasate from the vascular space more rapidly than usual or be sequestered in poorly perfused tissue. In such a case, the conditions required for the use of the dilution principle are not fulfilled, and accurate calculation of the blood volume cannot be made.

Measuring Other Body Spaces

Injection of a variety of tracers may be used to measure other volume spaces within the body. For example, sodium or potassium spaces may be measured using radioactive sodium and radioactive potassium. Labeled iodoantipyrine may be used to measure the body water volume. Such volume measurements are valid only if the concentration of tracer in the space sample accurately represents concentration throughout the entire volume.

A variety of other tracer techniques provide unique insight into a myriad of body metabolic functions. By these means, one can follow the course of iron through the body as it clears from the plasma, concentrates in the marrow, and reappears circulating in red cells. Alternatively, one can analyze the utilization of a labeled triglyceride by collecting and counting the radioactive carbon dioxide appearing in the breath after metabolism of the fat. These methods have provided unique tools for analyzing and increasing our understanding of a wide array of disease processes.

OTHER NONIMAGING QUANTITATIVE TESTS

Bone Densitometry

Osteoporosis is decreased bone content per unit volume of skeleton. It is a common condition associated with a number of processes and diseases. Because it exacts a large economic toll and causes significant morbidity and mortality in aging populations, osteoporosis constitutes an important public health problem. In addition to diseases that produce osteoporosis, risk factors for osteoporosis include female sex, aging, loss of estrogen secretion, Caucasian race, slender habitus, and delicate skeletal structures. Exogenous factors, such as exercise, alcohol, smoking, diet, and drugs, also affect the rate of bone loss. Conditions that interfere with alertness and ability to walk may provide the final provocation, leading to fall, fracture, and morbidity or mortality.

Since the prevalence of osteoporosis is high in these defined populations, some practitioners suggest prophylactic estrogen therapy for women with risk factors in spite of the documented increased risk of endometrial cancer associated with administration of estrogens. It seems rational that better objective measurements that could predict impending fracture associated with osteoporosis would better identify the population particularly at risk, thereby improving the risk/benefit ratio. There is, however, considerable controversy concerning the role of bone mineral measurement, particularly as an uncontrolled screening method, in defining a population appropriate for therapeutic intervention. This stems partly from the uneven distribution and progression of the osteoporotic process itself, the marked "normal" variation of bone mineral content, the relative newness of accurate and precise means for measuring bone mineral content, and even the uncertainty of the effectiveness of any therapy.

Measurement of Bone Mineral Content

Quantitative measurement of radiation transmitted through skeletal structures provides a unique means of measuring the mineral content of bone. The three most precise (reproducible) and accurate (actual correct measurement) techniques for quantitating bone mineral content include quantitative CT imaging (perferably using two different x-ray energies); single-photon absorptiometry, using a collimated beam of photons from a monoenergetic radioisotope source; dual-photon absorptiometry, using a radioisotope that emits photons of two different energies, and, more recently, use of a specially filtered x-ray beam which eliminates all but those x-ray energies appropriate for dual-photon absorptiometry.

The basic principle of measurement in all these techniques is the same; viz, the fraction of photons transmitted by tissue is related to the mass, density, and attenuation coefficient of that particular tissue for the particular photon energy being used. The attenuation coefficient, the fractional decrease in the number of photons passing through the tissue, is related to the energy of the photon and thus the kind of interaction it undergoes in tissue, the effective atomic number of the tissue and the electron density of the tissue. Attenuation coefficients may be expressed as lineal, related to the thickness of the tissue or in terms of mass related to the fractional decrease in photons per unit area density of the tissue. If the initial intensity of the radiation beam and its intensity after passing through tissue are known, mass characteristics of the tissue, such as its mineral content, can be calculated using the attenuation coefficients.

An important problem in measuring bone density at only one or two skeletal sites is that the osteoporotic process may have nonuniform distribution and effects. Early in the osteoporotic process, trabecular bone in the spine may be more affected than compact bone in the distal radius and weight-bearing bone may be affected differently. In part, this may reflect different rates of bone loss in trabecular as compared with cortical skeletal structures with aging and decreased estrogen levels. Interpretation of measurements must consider that individuals have variable rates of bone mass loss normally and in metabolic bone disease and that the rate of bone mass loss in an individual may not be constant.

Single-photon absorptiometry is restricted to sampling

appendicular skeleton with a preponderance of cortical bone except in the calcaneus, which is 99% trabecular bone. Dual-photon absorptiometry has the ability to sample a larger area of the skeleton, particularly the spine and the femoral neck, where trabecular bone predominates. The dual-photon technique permits mathematical correction for soft tissue absorption. Dual-photon absorptiometry also produces an image of the lumbar spine that may visualize atypical foci, such as large bone spurs, which contribute to a spurious estimation of bone mineral content. The dual-photon measurement process, however, is inherently more complex and requires stringent attention to calibration and control to ensure reproducibility. The same is true for quantitative CT imaging.

In a disease process requiring multiple measurements over a long period of time, reproducibility of the measurement itself is critical to the usefulness of the technique. In the hands of careful investigators, all these measurements can show excellent reproducibility. The considerations of cost and associated radiation favor the use of radioisotopes which deliver a fraction of the radiation dose associated with CT imaging and can be acquired at a fraction of the cost of a CT scanner. The dual-photon scanning technique using an x-ray beam and K–edge filters is also favorable for low radiation dose and cost. Such instruments can be dedicated to making bone mineral measurements.

It is apparent that serial bone mineral measurements may be valuable in selected individuals. In fact, these techniques are being used investigatively to document the direct relationship of bone mineral content to specific variables underlying osteoporosis as well as the effects of trial therapeutic interventions. However, it is also apparent that there are many unresolved problems in applying such techniques for large-scale screening. Some investigations indicate that the use of a simple reproducible measure of bone mineral mass may predict the likelihood of fracture occurrence. Further evaluation is necessary to establish the clinical efficacy of these procedures.

X-Ray Fluorescence

X-ray fluorescence is a tool for detecting and quantifying nonradioactive metals in a sample. Most often it is used to quantify the amount of iodine in blood, urine, or the thyroid gland. An americium-241 source irradiates the sample, emitting a 60-keV photon that interacts with an electron from the K shell of an iodine atom in the sample. This interaction results in emission of characteristic x-rays (28.5 and 32.4 keV for iodine), which are detected and measured by a semiconductor detector. The detector is interfaced to a computer that quantifies the characteristic x-rays produced and converts them into milligrams percent of iodine, based on previous measurements with known standards.

Other nonimaging procedures such as thyroid iodine uptake tests and fibrinogen uptake are discussed in Chapters 3 and 5. The underlying theme of all nuclear medicine tests—imaging and nonimaging—is quantification. Through quantitative analyses of imaging and nonimaging data, nuclear medicine provides functional evaluations of body physiology, biochemistry, and metabolism.

SELECTED READINGS

Radioligand Assays

Berson SA, Yalow R. Immunoassay of an endogenous plasma insulin in man. *J Clin Invest* 1960; 39:1115–1175

Goldsmith SJ. Radioimmunoassay: Review of basic principles. *Semin Nucl Med* 1975; 5:125–152

Kirchner PT (ed). Radioassay. In: *Nuclear medicine review syllabus.* New York: Society of Nuclear Medicine; 1980:491–538

Moss AJ Jr, Dalrymple GV, Boyd CM. *Practical radioimmunoassay.* St. Louis: CV Mosby; 1976

Thorell JI, Larson SN. *Radioimmunoassay and related techniques.* St. Louis: CV Mosby; 1978

Schilling Test

Fairbanks VF, Wahner HW, Phyliky RL. Tests for pernicious anemia: The "Schilling test." *Mayo Clin Proc* 1983; 58:541–544

Measuring Body Spaces

Wright RR, Tono M, Pollycove M. Blood volume. *Semin Nucl Med* 1975; 5:63–78

Bone Mineral Measurements

Cameron JR, Mazess RB, Sorenson JA. Precision and accuracy of bone mineral determination by direct photon absorptiometry. *Invest Radiol* 1968; 3:141–150

Genant HK, Ettinger B, Cann CE, et al. Osteoporosis: assessment by quantitative computed tomography. *Orthop Clin North Am* 1985; 16:557–568

Richelson LS, Wahner HW, Melton LJ III, Riggs BL. Relative contribution of aging and estrogen deficiency to postmenopausal bone loss. *N Engl J Med* 1984; 311:1273–1275

Riggs BL, Melton LJ III. Involutional osteoporosis. *N Engl J Med* 1986; 314:1676–1686

Riggs BL, Wahner HW, Jeeman E, et al. Changes in bone mineral density of the proximal femur and spine with aging. *J Clin Invest* 1982; 70:716–723

Wahner HW. Assessment of metabolic bone disease: Review of new nuclear medicine procedures. *Mayo Clin Proc* 1985; 60:827–835

Wasnich RD, Ross PD, Heilbrun LK, Vogel JM. Prediction of postmenopausal fracture risk with use of bone mineral measurements. *Am J Obstet Gynecol* 1985; 153:745–751

Appendix and Glossary

Appendix: Sensitivities and Specificities of Nuclear Medicine Tests

Disease or Physiologic State	Appropriate Radionuclide Study	Sensitivity	Specificity	Comments
Cardiopulmonary disease				
Ischemic heart disease	Stress thallium study	High to very high	Very high	—
	Rest and stress gated imaging ejection fraction	High to very high	Moderate	—
Acute myocardial infarction	Rest thallium study	Very high	Moderate	Best done within 12–24 hr; cannot distinguish old from new infarct; expensive
	Pyrophosphate imaging	Moderately high	Moderate	Best for transmural infarction between 24–72 hr

Appendix: Sensitivities and Specificities of Nuclear Medicine Tests

Disease or Physiologic State	Appropriate Radionuclide Study	Sensitivity	Specificity	Comments
Pulmonary embolus	Ventilation/perfusion imaging	Very high	Moderately high	Specificity varies according to ventilation abnormalities
Bronchial obstructive disease	Xenon-133 gas washout	Very high	Moderate	Defines physiology
Interstitial lung disease	Gallium-67 imaging or DTPA washout	High for active disease	Low	—
Gastrointestinal and liver disease				
Esophageal motility	Radionuclide esophageal transit	High	Low	—
Gastroesophageal reflux	Radionuclide quantitative reflux study	Very high	High	—
Gastric emptying	Labeled solid and liquid meals	Very high	Low	—

Condition	Test			Can be used to document occult aspiration
Pulmonary aspiration of gastric contents	Technetium-99m colloid administered orally	Uncertain	High	Can be used to document occult aspiration
Blind loop syndrome	Bile acid breath test	High	—	—
Pancreatic insufficiency	Tripalmitin breath test	High	Moderate	—
GI bleeding (lower)	Technetium-99m colloid	Very high (compared with angiography)	High	Detects only active bleeding
GI bleeding (intermittent and/or acute active)	Technetium-99m red cells	High	Moderate	—
Ectopic gastric mucosa	Pertechnetate imaging	High	Moderate	—
Alcoholic liver disease	Liver scan	Moderate	Low	—
Diffuse hepatocellular disease	Liver scan	Moderate	Low	—
Hepatic abscess	Liver scan	Moderate	Low	—

Appendix: Sensitivities and Specificities of Nuclear Medicine Tests

Disease or Physiologic State	Appropriate Radionuclide Study	Sensitivity	Specificity	Comments
Cholecystitis (acute)	HIDA study	Very high	Very high	—
Bile reflux	HIDA study	Very high	Moderate	—
Skeletal–joint and muscle				
Paget's disease	Bone scan	High	Low	—
Hypertrophic osteoar- thropathy	Bone scan	High	Moderate	—
Hyperparathy- roidism	Diphosphonate retention	Moderate	Moderate	—
Rheumatoid arthritis	Bone scan	High	Low	—
Fracture	Bone scan	High	Low	—
Infarct	Bone scan	High	Low	Specificity high for 24 hr and low thereafter

Osteoporosis				
Single- and dual-photon absorptiometry		High	—	Efficacy as screening procedure to be determined
Dermatomyositis and rhabdomyolysis	Bone scan	Moderate	Moderate	Visualizes ongoing myocytolysis
Endocrinologic disease				
Thyroid status	T_3, T_4, TSH by RIA	Very high	High	—
Thyroid nodules	Thyroid scan	Moderate	Low	—
Thyroiditis	Thyroid scan	Moderate	Low	—
Acute or subacute thyroiditis	RAI uptake	Moderate	Low	—
Hashimoto's thyroiditis	RAI uptake with perchlorate washout	Moderate	High	—
Hyperparathyroidism	Thallium-pertechnetate subtraction imaging	High	Moderate	Use to locate abnormal tissue

Appendix: Sensitivities and Specificities of Nuclear Medicine Tests

Disease or Physiologic State	Appropriate Radionuclide Study	Sensitivity	Specificity	Comments
Cushing's syndrome caused by adrenal adenoma or hyperplasia	Adrenal scan with suppression	High	High	—
Pheochromocytoma	Metaiodobenzylguanidine imaging	High	High	—
Infectious diseases				
Bacteremia	Radioactive CO_2 production by bacteria in culture	High	High	Positive sooner than standard culture
Abdominal abscess including subphrenic	Gallium imaging	Moderate	Low	—
Pyelonephritis	Labeled WBC	High	High	—
	Gallium	Moderate	Moderate	—

Cerebral herpes	Brain scan	High	Low	May be positive before CT findings
Cerebral abscess	Brain scan	High	Low	—
Hematologic disorders				
Hemolytic disorders	Red cell survival and sequestration	High	High	Usually unnecessary
Marrow failure	Iron blood clearance and marrow uptake	High	Moderate	Usually unnecessary
Pernicious anemia	Schilling test	Very high	Very high	Differentiates various causes of B_{12} malabsorption
Neoplastic disease				
Metastatic disease	Liver imaging in lung, GI, and breast neoplasms	High	Low	—
	Skeletal imaging in breast, lung, and prostate	High	Moderate	—

Appendix: Sensitivities and Specificities of Nuclear Medicine Tests

Disease or Physiologic State	Appropriate Radionuclide Study	Sensitivity	Specificity	Comments
Lung cancer	Gallium imaging	Moderate	Low	Helpful noninvasive staging
Differentiated thyroid cancer	TBG by RIA	High	Moderate	—
	Iodine-131 whole-body imaging	High	Moderate	Liver, stomach, and residual thyroid are imaged
Genitourinary disease				
Renal clearance	Iodine-125 iothalamate and Technetium-99m DTPA imaging	Not applicable	Not applicable	—
Renal vascular problems	Technetium-99m DTPA angiogram and transit curves;	High	—	Accuracy may be enhanced by use of captopril

Condition	Test			
Renal mass	Iodine-131 or ^{123}I hippuran images and renogram; Technetium-99m MAG$_3$ renogram and images	High	Low	—
Asymmetric renal function	Technetium-99m DMSA, gluco-heptonate, imaging	High	Moderate	Helpful in renovascular hypertension
	Technetium-99m DMSA imaging	High	Moderate	—
Obstructive uropathy	Hippuran renogram; Diuretic renogram using hippuran or ^{99m}Tc DTPA with furosemide	High	High	—
Reflux	Voiding cystogram	Very high	Very high	—
Spermatic cord torsion	Scrotal imaging	High	Moderate	—

Appendix: Sensitivities and Specificities of Nuclear Medicine Tests

Disease or Physiologic State	Appropriate Radionuclide Study	Sensitivity	Specificity	Comments
Central nervous system disease				
Cerebral death	Cerebral radionuclide perfusion study	Very high	Very high	—
Cerebrovascular disease	Xenon washout	High	High	—
	Technetium-99m cerebral angiogram	Moderate	Moderate	—
	Technetium-99m HMPAO, IMP–I–123 imaging	Very high	—	Still experimental
Normal pressure hydrocephalus	Cisternography	Not well defined	See discussion in Chapter 13, Radionuclide Cisternography	
CSF leak	Cisternography	Very high	Very high	Requires LP

Vascular disease

Trauma to moderately large arteries	Radionuclide angiogram	High	Moderate	—
Thrombophlebitis	Iodine-125 fibrinogen uptake	High in calves	Moderate	—
Venous occlusive disease	Radionuclide venogram	Moderate	Moderate	—
Atheromata	Indium-111 platelet imaging	Under evaluation	—	—

Abbreviations: CSF, cerebrospinal fluid; CT, computed tomography; DMSA, dimethylsuccinic acid; DTPA, diethylenetriaminepentaacetic acid; GI, gastrointestinal; HIDA, hepatobiliary iminodiacetic acid; RAIU, radioactive iodide uptake; RIA, radioimmunoassay; TBG, thyroxine-binding globulin; T_3, triiodothyronine; T_4, thyroxine; TSH, thyroid-stimulating hormone; WBC, white blood cells.

Glossary

Absorbed dose: Energy absorbed per unit mass of irradiated tissue; a rad is the unit of absorbed dose that signifies absorption of 100 erg/g. SI unit: the gray; 1 Gy = 1 j/kg = 100 rad.

Absorption: Transfer of energy from incident radiation to tissue.

Aerosol scan: Use of a nebulized radioactive mist deposited in the lung airways to form an image.

Aggregated albumin: Albumin denatured under specific pH and heat conditions to yield friable particles of certain sizes; macroaggregates of albumin (MAA) 25–50 μm in diameter are used for temporary arteriolar capillary blockade, for example, in perfusion lung imaging. Microaggregates <300 nm in diameter are used to study reticuloendothelial function.

Albumin microspheres: Microspheres of albumin 40–60 μm in diameter produced under specific conditions of heat and pH in oil, used for temporary arteriolar capillary blockade.

Alpha (α) decay: Emission of a positively charged helium nucleus from an unstable nucleus.

Alpha (α)-particle: A helium nucleus, two protons, and two neutrons.

Amplification: Boosting of electronic signals produced by ionizing radiation to make them measurable.

Analog data: Nondigital information that is continuously variable; film recording is an analog means of data storage.

Analyzer: An instrument for discriminating energy levels of detected radiation.

203

Anger camera: Instrument invented by Hal Anger, for recording distribution of γ-emitting radioactivity in the body; it can detect radiation over its entire face, which ranges from 25 to 52.5 cm in diameter. Also called scintillation camera and gamma camera.

Angiography: Recording of the transit of an imageable substance through a vessel by means of a rapid sequence of images.

Annihilation radiation: Energy produced when a positron interacts with an electron. The particles disappear, and two γ-rays of 511-keV energy each are emitted at 180° to one another.

Anode: Electrode maintained at a relatively positive potential.

Artifact: A spurious structure or feature in an image or data produced by the imaging technique or instrument rather than by the imaged object itself.

Atom: The smallest divisible component of matter that maintains characteristic, unique properties of an element.

Atomic mass: Atomic weight in atomic mass units.

Atomic mass number (symbol A): Sum of the number of protons, the atomic number symbolized by Z, and the number of neutrons, symbolized by N, in the nucleus.

Atomic mass unit: A unit of mass equal to $\frac{1}{12}$ the mass of a carbon-12 atom: 1 amu = 1.6605×10^{-27} kg; electron = 0.00055 amu; proton = 1.00727 amu; neutron = 1.00866 amu.

Atomic number (symbol Z): Number of protons in the nucleus; it determines the number of orbital electrons and hence the chemical properties of an atom.

Atomic weight (at wt): The mass of a neutral atom relative to carbon as 12.000; thus expressed, the weight of the atom in amu to the nearest integer is equal to its mass number, A.

Attenuation: Reduction of radiation intensity as it passes through matter in which the radiation is absorbed or scattered.

Attenuation coefficient: Fraction of the incident beam of photons removed by a material. The lineal coefficient is the fraction absorbed per unit thickness. The mass coefficient is the fraction absorbed per unit area density.

Auger electron: An orbital electron emitted from the atom and carrying the energy, as an alternative to characteristic x-ray emission.

Autofluoroscope: Camera composed of a mosaic of 294 crystals arranged in rectangular (14 × 21) rank and file, the outputs of which are fed directly into computer core memory; data are stored and retrieved in digital form.

Autonomous nodule: A thyroid nodule that functions independently of thyroid-stimulating hormone.

Autoradiograph: Deposition of silver grains by interaction of radiation contained in tissue placed in intimate contact with photographic emulsion, producing a record of the distribution of radioactivity.

Average life: The average lifetime of an atom of a particular radionuclide before undergoing radioactive decay, equal to 1.44 times the half-life of the radionuclide.

Background radiation: Ubiquitous radiation present in varying amounts in varying locations caused by surroundings, natural or otherwise.

Baseline: Refers to the discriminator setting that determines the lowest-energy photon that will be counted or recorded.

Bayes' theorem: Theorem relating the probability of, for example, the presence or absence of a disease after a certain test is performed, to the probability of its presence or absence before performing the test.

Becquerel (Bq): The Système Internationale (SI) unit of activity, equal to 1 disintegration per second (dps): megabecquerel (MBq) = 10^6 dps = 27.03 microcuries (μCi); gigabecquerel (GBq) = 10^9 dps = 27.03 millicuries (mCi).

Beta (β)-particle: An energetic (high-speed) electron emitted from an unstable nucleus.

Bile acid breath test: Test that measures the presence of gut bacteria deconjugating a bile acid; radioactive CO_2 in the breath is collected and measured after administration of a C-14-radiolabeled bile acid.

Blood-brain barrier: Peculiarity of exchange between the brain and plasma solutes related to tight capillary endothelial junctions in the brain.

Brain scan: Images of the cranium and its contents in which normal brain does not concentrate intravenously injected radioactivity.

Breath test: One of a group of tests in which metabolism of a compound labeled with ^{14}C, usually at a terminal carboxyl group, is measured by the amount of labeled CO_2 excreted in the breath.

Bremsstrahlung (German for "braking radiation"): Continuous spectrum of electromagnetic energy produced by collisions between β-particles or other high-speed electrons and atomic nuclei; qualitatively identical to x-rays and γ-rays.

Camera: See Anger camera.

Camera, positron: Device for detecting and quantitating distribution of positron-emitting radionuclides in the body.

Capillary blockade: Blockage of a fraction of a capillary bed by metabolizable particles (aggregated albumin) injected downstream from the capillary bed.

Carbon-11: A 20-min half-life positron-emitting radioactive carbon; used with CO or CO_2 to derive cardiopulmonary information and in other applications requiring carbon-labeled imaging agents.

Carbon-14: A 5730-year half-life, pure β-emitter used in various synthesized fatty acid compounds and bile acids for breath test absorption studies, for hormone radioassay, and as an indicator for metabolic cycles; cannot be counted in the body.

Carrier: Nonradioactive element or compound with the same chemical properties as the radioactive labeled molecule. The carrier undergoes the process being studied.

Carrier-free: Composed solely of a single isotopic species.

Cathode: The relatively negatively charged electrode.

Characteristic radiation: Radiation of a particular frequency or energy emitted during transition of electrons from one atomic shell to another.

Cisternography: Delineation of the cerebrospinal fluid spaces surrounding the brain after intrathecal instillation of a suitable radiopharmaceutical.

Coincidence counting: Counting of the simultaneously occurring annihilation γ-rays resulting from positron–electron interaction.

Collimator: The heavy metal barrier with fixed geometrically arranged holes to permit passage of γ-rays traveling only in certain paths to reach the crystal detector; it geometrically defines the field to which the detector is sensitive.

Colloid: Suspension of particles 10–500 nm (nanometers) in diameter used because they are phagocytized by reticuloendothelial cells.

Competitive protein binding assay: See Radioimmunoassay.

Compton scatter: A process in which an x-ray or γ-ray is deflected by collision with an electron; the x-ray or γ-ray loses energy in the process, which is transferred in the collision to the electron.

Computed tomography: Use of a computer and data from either x-rays, radionuclides, or nuclear magnetic resonance to produce body section images. These calculated images represent the following: *x-ray (CT):* tissue densities from absorption coefficients when x-rays are transmitted; *radionuclide emission computed tomography (ECT):* origin of emitted photons when radionuclides are administered and photons emitted; *magnetic resonance imaging (MRI):* tissue T_1 and T_2 values, as well as quantities of magnetically polar nuclei such as hydrogen, which emit a characteristic resonant frequency in a uniform, graded magnetic field when excited by radiofrequency.

Contamination: Accidental spread of unwanted radioactivity to an area where it does not belong.

Contrast enhancement: The exaggeration of small differences in count rate distribution by large differences in density on a recording medium such as film; the process permits ready visual perception of small differences in distribution that would not be apparent using linear data representation.

Contrast media: Compounds used to produce density differences in tissues, organs, or vessels to permit their imaging. X-ray contrast media are largely iodinated organic molecules that are either selectively excreted by a particular organ after intravenous injection or are injected intravascularly; their high iodine content strongly absorbs x-rays and attenuates the beam.

Conversion electron: An energetic electron emitted from an electron orbit carrying the energy from a nuclear transition; an alternative to γ-ray emission.

Cosmic radiation: Radiation consisting of high-energy particles (chiefly atomic nuclei) that originates from outer space, and showers of particles and electromagnetic radiation produced when they bombard the earth's atmosphere.

Count: The detected number of events from radioactive disintegrations.

Count rate: The detected number of events per unit time from radioactive disintegrations.

Counting statistics: In counting radioactivity, this refers to statistical variability of counts or count rate.

Cow: Colloquial term; see Generator.

Critical organ: The organ or tissue that receives the largest dose of radiation in a procedure. This depends on radionuclide concentration by the organ, geometric factors, and the effective retention in that organ.

Crystal, scintillation: A crystalline solid, such as sodium iodide containing trace amounts of thallium activator NaI(Tl), which emits light scintillation when it absorbs ionizing radiation; essentially transforms invisible electromagnetic radiation or particles into visible photons.

CT: See Computed tomography.

Curie (Ci): The quantity of radioactivity having 3.7×10^{10} disintegrations per second: mCi = millicurie = 10^{-3} curie; μCi = microcurie = 10^{-6} curie; 1 millicurie = 37 megabecquerel.

"Cutie pie": (Colloquial) Portable ionization chamber for determining relatively stable dose rates.

Cyclotron: Device used to accelerate charged particles maintained in a spiral trajectory electromagnetically; the resultant high-energy particle may be used to irradiate targets to produce radioactive substances.

Daughter: See Generator.

Deadtime: The period after detecting a radiation event during which the detector cannot respond to another event.

Decay constant (λ): The fraction of radioactive nuclei undergoing decay per unit time.

Decay, radioactive: The spontaneous transformation of an energetic unstable nucleus to one of lower energy accompanied by the emission of high-energy photons or particles.

Detector: A device used to measure radioactivity.

Digital autofluoroscope: See Autofluoroscope.

Digital recording system: A system in which detected events are stored as numbers.

Digital subtraction angiography: Technique that uses computer-enhanced video images to display vascular opacification after intravenous or intra-arterial administration of contrast media.

Discriminator: See Analyzer.

Disintegration: See Decay, radioactive.

Disk: Ferric-coated disk on which information may be stored in magnetic tracks and rapidly read in a fashion similar conceptually to a phonograph record.

DMSA: Dimethylsuccinic acid, a renal cortical imaging agent.

Dose: See Absorbed dose.

Dose equivalent (H): A special quantity used in radiation protection and radiation risk estimation, equal to the product of the absorbed dose D in rads, times the quality factor Q for the type of radiation involved, times any other dose-modifying factors to account for special radiation sensitivity of the irradiated tissue; the basic unit of dose equivalent is the rem (SI unit: the sievert, $1\ Sv = 100\ rem$).

Dosimeter: Device used to measure the amount of radiation exposure or dose received.

Dosimetry: Measurement or calculation of delivered radiation dose.

DTPA: Diethylenetriaminepentaacetic acid; a chelating agent that is excreted from the plasma via glomerular filtration when complexed with a variety of atoms such as technetium-99m, chromium-51, or indium-111.

Dynamic images: A series of rapidly obtained sequential images depicting a rapidly changing physiologic event such as regional perfusion.

Dynode: One of a series of electrodes that, held at sequentially higher potentials, multiplies bombarding electrons in stages of a photomultiplier tube.

ECT (emission computed tomography): Technique that uses a computer to reconstruct in a variety of planes (transaxial, coronal, sagittal) the distribution of a radiopharmaceutical within the body as imaged by a scintillation camera.

Efficiency, detection: The ratio of detected to incident or total events.

Ejection fraction: In cardiac studies refers to the ratio of ventricular stroke volume to ventricular end-diastolic volume; provides an index of ventricular function.

Electromagnetic radiation: Electrical and magnetic energy in the form of waves or packets of energy called photons traveling through space at the speed of light; the spectrum of electromagnetic radiation ranges from long-wavelength, low-energy radiowaves to very high-energy, short-wavelength x-rays and γ-rays.

Electron: Fundamental negatively charged particle.

Electron capture: Nuclear decay by interaction of the nucleus with an orbital electron in which the electron is captured by the nucleus with subsequent emission of a neutrino and characteristic x-ray and decrease of the atomic number.

Electron volt (eV): Energy acquired by 1 electron accelerated across a potential difference of 1 volt = 1.6×10^{-12} erg: keV = kiloelectron volt = 1.6×10^{-9} erg; MeV = megaelectron volt = 1.6×10^{-6} erg.

Emission computed tomography: See ECT.

Emission scan: Image formed by external detection of radiation emitted from internally administered radioactivity, as opposed to external radiation transmitted through the area of interest.

Energy: The capacity for doing work; nuclear energy results from the equivalence of mass and energy according to the relationship stated by Einstein, $E = mc^2$.

Equilibrium, radioactive: A state in which isotopic production by a parent nuclear species equals its loss by disintegration of the daughter product species.

Excitation: The addition of energy to a system rendering it unstable and likely to give off the excess energy spontaneously.

Exposure: Quantity referring to the amount of ionization produced by x-rays or γ-rays as they pass through air, used to specify environmental radiation levels; can be measured with ionization chambers; basic unit is the roentgen (1 R = 2.58×10^{-4} coulombs/kg air).

Field of view: the region "seen" by a detector crystal; it defines the volume from which emitted activity may be detected.

Fluorescence scanning: Imaging process in which atoms are excited by impinging external radiation of an energy near the binding energy of the orbital electrons; the removal of the orbital electron results in characteristic x-ray production that may then be detected by a suitable semiconductor detector linked to the exciting source; used to map iodine distribution in the thyroid using americium-241 as the excitation source.

Fluorine-18: A positron-emitting radioisotope of fluorine with a half-life of 110 min.

Focal plane: Theoretic plane defined by the geometric convergence of the collimator holes.

Focused collimator: Collimator with holes that geometrically converge in space in front of the collimator.

Fourier transform: Mathematical treatment of spatially or temporally varying data that considers frequency variations as the sum of a number of sine/cosine functions. Used in tomographic image reconstruction (CT, ECT, MRI) and for analyzing temporally varying data, such as cardiac chamber volume changes.

Frequency: Number of cycles per measured unit of time or distance; 1 hertz (Hz) = $1 \ sec^{-1}$.

Frequency, radiation (ν): Number of complete phase cycles per second of an electromagnetic radiation treated as a wave function, which is related directly to the photon energy by Planck's constant, h, in the formula $E = h\nu$.

Frequency response curve: The data output curve from an imaging system in response to input of varying spatial or temporal frequency.

Gamma camera: See Anger camera.

Gamma (γ) ray: Electromagnetic radiation emitted from the nucleus of a decaying radionuclide

Gated image: An image made from data acquired only over a brief selected physiologic interval, usually a selected portion of the cardiac cycle, such as end-systole or end-diastole; the image data acquisition is triggered or gated by the R wave for short 10–40-msec periods at a selected interval or intervals from the R wave to coincide with end-systole (downslope of T wave) and end-diastole (R wave itself); sufficient cycles are repetitively gated to build up data for a diagnostic image.

Gaussian distribution (normal distribution): A mathematical function describing the distribution of events in terms of the mean and standard deviation of the population or events under observation; produces a bell-shaped curve when plotted graphically.

Geiger-Müller tube: A gas-filled tube with collecting electrode (anode) maintained at high voltage to collect, multiply, and measure the ions produced by entering ionizing radiation.

Generator: A column filled with a long-half-life parent radionuclide that decays to a short-half-life daughter nuclide which then can be separated by physical or chemical means.

Gigabecquerel (GBq): That quantity of radioactivity exhibiting 10^9 disintegrations per second.

Genetically significant dose: That radiation dose which, if received by every member of a defined population, would be expected to produce the same total genetic injury to the population as do the actual doses received by its various individuals.

Geometry: Refers to the geometric relationship between the detector and activity to be measured which determines the fraction of total emitted radiation that can be detected.

Gray (Gy): SI unit of absorbed dose: 1 Gy = 1 j/kg = 100 rad.

Ground state: Lowest energy level that can be attained in a nucleus of given configuration.

Half-life: The time required for a decaying substance to reach half its initial value; *biologic* refers to the time for the body or an organ to eliminate one-half the original material; *physical* refers to physical radioactive decay of nuclei to one-half their original numbers; *effective* refers to the combined effects of biologic elimination and physical decay, which results in an observed half-life shorter than either of these two values individually.

Half-value layer (HVL): The thickness of a material that attenuates an incident beam of electromagnetic radiation by one-half.

Heavy particles: Neutrons and charged particles with a mass of 1 or greater.

HIDA: Hepatobiliary imaging agents with substituted carbamoyl moiety linked to iminodiacetic acid.

Hippuran: See Iodohippurate.

Human albumin microspheres: See Albumin microspheres.

IDA: Agents containing iminodiacetic acid for hepatobiliary imaging; see HIDA.

Information density: The number of counts recorded per unit area of the object being imaged; a sufficient information density must be achieved to obviate the effects of statistical fluctuation on image quality.

Internal conversion: Process in which energy from an excited nucleus is transferred to one of its orbital electrons, which is then emitted from the atom.

Iodohippurate (Hippuran): Orthoiodohippurate salt excreted by the kidneys chiefly through tubular secretion with ~80% efficiency and used to measure effective renal plasma flow. About 20% is excreted by glomerular filtration, 80% via tubular secretion.

Ion: A charged particle; atoms or groups of atoms that have gained or lost electrons and consequently carry a charge.

Ionization chamber: A gas-filled chamber with electrodes maintained at a potential difference to collect and measure current attributable to ion pairs produced by incident radiation.

Ionizing radiation: Radiation that produces ion pairs as it passes through matter.

Isobar: Nuclides with the same mass number, but different atomic numbers.

Isomer: Nuclides having the same mass and atomic numbers but different energy states for a measurable period of time.

Isomeric transition: Transition of nuclear isomer to a lower energy state, for example, technetium-99m decays to technetium-99.

Isotope: Nuclides having the same atomic number and hence the same chemical properties, but different mass numbers; for example, ^{131}I and ^{127}I are isotopes of iodine.

K shell: Inner orbital electron path adjacent to the nucleus.

Kiloelectron-volt (keV): One thousand electronvolts.

Krypton-81m: Short, 13-sec-half-life radionuclide of the inert gas krypton, which can be obtained from a Rb-81/Kr-81m generator and used in studying lung ventilation.

L shell: The second electron orbital path from the nucleus.

Labeled compound: A compound joined to a radioactive indicator.

Linear energy transfer (LET): The energy transferred by ionizing radiation to the target atoms per unit distance of penetration; the number of ionizations produced along the particle track is a function of particle charge and velocity.

Liquid scintillation counter: A device used principally for counting β-particles; the material containing a β-emitter is dissolved or suspended in a liquid which, when excited by the β-emission, in turn emits light (scintillations) that can be detected.

Lymphoscintigraphy: Functional imaging of a regional lymphatic system obtained by injecting a radioactive minicolloid into the soft tissue drained by that system.

Macroaggregated albumin (MAA): See Aggregated albumin.

Magnetic resonance imaging (MRI): See Nuclear magnetic resonance.

Mass number: See Atomic mass number; see Atomic weight.

Maximum permissible dose (MPD): Guidelines for the maximum amount of radiation that may be received by an individual working with radiation within a specified time period; for those in occupations dealing with radiation MPD (rems) = 5 rem/year.

Mean transit time: The time it takes the average indicator population to traverse a defined volume; when multiplied by the average height of the curve, it equals the area under curve of counts versus time generated as the indicator traverses a designated volume.

Megabecquerel (MBq): That quantity of radioactivity having 10^6 disintegrations per second.

Metastable state: An unstable nuclear state having a finite and measurable lifetime that decays to a more stable state by γ-emission without change in the atomic number; abbreviated by the letter m.

Microcurie (μCi): That quantity of radioactivity exhibiting 3.7×10^4 disintegrations per second.

Million electron-volts (MeV): 10^6 eV.

Millirad (mrad): 10^{-3} rad.

Millirem (mrem): 10^{-3} rem.

Minicolloid: Radioactive colloid with particle sizes averaging 10 nanometers (nm) in diameter, usually formulated with antimony and used for evaluating lymphatic drainage.

Modulation transfer function (MTF): A mathematical function describing the ability of an imaging system to reproduce line patterns of varying spatial frequency (lines or line pairs per centimeter) in an image.

Molybdenum-99: The relatively long-half-life parent, 65 hr, of technetium-99m, used to make Mo-99–Tc-99m generators.

MUGA study: See Multiple gated acquisition study.

Multichannel analyzer: An electronic device for sorting photons of different energies according to energy levels.

Multiple gated acquisition study (MUGA study): Study of cardiac contractility and wall motion. The blood pool is rendered radioactive; the cardiac cycle is divided into many (usually 16–32, but can be more) equal time intervals from R wave to R wave, and counts from each interval are stored as they are recorded in computer frames corresponding to each interval; each R wave triggers the acquisition process again until sufficient data are built up in each frame to form a diagnostic image. Multiple (16–32) images are formed, processed, and displayed in cine format. Ejection fractions from individual cardiac chambers, as well as other indices of cardiac function, can be derived.

Nanocurie (nCi): 10^{-9} curies; that amount of radioactivity having 37 disintegrations per second.

Neutrino: A particle emitted from the nucleus with no electrical charge and virtually no mass that carries energy in β-decay and electron-capture processes; not detectable by conventional radiation detectors.

Neutron: An elementary particle of mass 1.00866 amu having no charge.

Nuclear magnetic resonance: A means of detecting atoms having a net magnetic moment by placing them in a uniform magnetic field and inducing characteristic resonant frequency with an appropriate external radiofrequency current; the characteristic resonant frequency may then be detected; such a system may be used to produce sectional body images of molecular distributions, particularly of hydrogen. For imaging, also called magnetic resonance imaging (MRI).

Nuclear reactor: A device for producing controlled fission that yields neutrons and energy from fissionable material; fission in reactors produces radionuclides used in medical practice; neutrons are also used to bombard stable targets to produce radionuclides.

Nucleide: Refers to a nucleic acid.

Nucleon: Nuclear constituent particles; neutrons, and protons.

Nucleotide: Refers to a phosphorylated nucleic acid.

Nuclide: An individual nuclear species uniquely characterized by atomic number (Z) and atomic mass (A).

Pair production: Conversion of electromagnetic radiation greater than 1.02 MeV in energy in a nuclear field into an electron and a positron.

Penetration: Piercing of detector shielding or collimator septa by γ-rays; contributes to image degradation.

Pertechnetate (TcO_4^-): The form in which technetium-99m is obtained from commonly available generators; the technetium in this molecule may be reduced and made reactive to label a variety of other compounds.

PET (positron emission computed tomography): Formation of tomographic images of the distribution in the body of compounds labeled with positron emitters; the use of positrons that emit detectable annihilation radiation at 180° and special paired detectors permits quantitation of the compound distribution; computer reconstruction of data obtained from 360° around the body permits reconstruction by suitable algorithms of two-dimensional cross sections of the positron distribution in the body.

Phantom: A volume of material that has physical absorption and transmission characteristics of tissue and hence may be used to simulate the human body tissue. Also refers to a container for radioactivity often made in the shape of an organ and used to study instrument resolution.

Phosphonates: Phosphate analogs with a P—C—P linkage replacing the P—O—P linkage; they may be labeled with technetium-99m and serve as bone imaging agents.

Photoelectric effect: Interaction of electromagnetic radiation with matter involving bound electrons; the electromagnetic radiation is completely absorbed by the atom that then ejects a bound electron with kinetic energy equal to the difference between the absorbed electromagnetic energy and the binding energy of the ejected electron; a characteristic x-ray (or Auger electron) is subsequently produced when the vacated shell is filled by another orbital electron.

Photomultiplier tube: Electronic tube that converts light flashes to electrons and then multiplies the electrons in dynode stages, resulting in a detectable pulse of electrical current.

Photon: Specifically refers to particle-like behavior of electromagnetic radiation; the quantum of electromagnetic energy having no mass or charge but possessing a discrete amount of energy.

Photoscan: Film recording of radioisotope distribution from a rectilinear scanning device.

Pinhole collimator: Heavy metal collimator operating on the geometric principle of a pinhole camera; the image of a small object close to the pinhole is inverted and magnified as the virtual image passes through the small pinhole across a relatively large distance to the detector surface.

PIPIDA: One of the IDA agents for hepatobiliary imaging; see IDA.

Poisson distribution: A mathematical distribution that describes probability of radioactive decay; the standard deviation of the mean number of events N, is $\sqrt{N}$; for large numbers of discrete events, the Poisson distribution is approximated by the gaussian or normal distribution.

Positron: A particle with the mass of an electron and a unit positive charge.

Positron emission computed tomography: See PET.

Proton: Hydrogen nucleus with a mass number of 1, a positive charge of 1 and a mass of 1.00727 amu; the number of protons in the nucleus Z establishes the chemical properties of an atom.

Pulse-height analyzer: An instrument capable of separating out pulses produced by absorbed photons of different energy levels according to the voltage height of the pulse produced.

Quality control: Procedures performed to determine that a radiopharmaceutical has appropriate physical and chemical properties or that an instrument is operating properly.

Quality factor (Q): Factor by which the absorbed dose D in rads is multiplied to obtain the dose equivalent H in rems; the value depends specifically on the ionization density, LET, produced by the radiation. For x-, γ-, and β-radiation, $Q = 1$. For heavy particles such as neutrons and α-particles $Q = 10$–20.

Rad: Unit of measurement for absorbed radiation dose; 1 rad imparts 100 erg/g to the absorbing medium.

Radiation dose: See Absorbed dose, Dose equivalent, Rad, and Rem.

Radioactivity: Spontaneous disintegration of an unstable nucleus with emission of either energetic particles or electromagnetic radiation or both.

Radioaerosol: Radioactive compound nebulized into an aerosol for inhalation.

Radioactive iodine uptake (RAIU): See Thyroid uptake.

Radiocolloid: A radioactive substance in colloidal form.

Radiograph: An image produced by recording transmitted x-rays on so-called x-ray film.

Radioimmunoassay (RIA): An assay using competition between a radiolabeled antigen and the same antigen in the serum for antibody binding sites; during equilibrium, the more unlabeled serum antigen present, the less radiolabeled antigen will be bound to the antibody; the serum level is measured by determining the bound:free ratio it produces compared with known standards in the same system.

Radioisotope: A radioactive member of an isotope family; for example, iodine-131 is a radioisotope of iodine.

Radionuclide: Refers specifically to a radioactive nuclide. For example, iodine-131 is a radionuclide, whereas iodine-127 is a stable nuclide.

Radiopharmaceutical: A radionuclide or compound labeled with radioactivity used for a diagnostic purpose or a local physical effect for a therapeutic outcome rather than a pharmacologic effect.

Radiotracer: (see Tracer) A radioactive tracer.

RAIU: Radioactive iodine uptake; see Thyroid uptake.

Ratemeter: An instrument that detects and displays a time-averaged count rate of radioactivity viewed by a detector.

Rectilinear scanner: Instrument for detecting distribution of radioactivity by moving back and forth over the area of interest and recording detected activity in serial strips until the entire area is imaged.

Reflux study: In gastroenterology, a study done to document reflux of gastric contents into the esophagus; in urology, a study done to document reflux of a substance instilled in the bladder into the upper urinary tract.

Relative biologic effectiveness (RBE): A concept used in experimental radiobiology to relate the amount of radiation dose required in two different experimental situations or for two different types of radiation to obtain a specified biologic end point (e.g., a certain percentage of cells killed in a cell culture); generally taken as the ratio of dose of x-rays or γ-rays required under standardized conditions to that required for the tested radiation and conditions.

Rem: Unit of dose equivalent, used specifically for radiation protection and risk estimation, obtained by multiplying the absorbed dose D in rads by the quality factor Q for the particular type of radiation involved, and by any other dose-modifying factors; dose-modifying factors may be included for tissues that are especially sensitive to radiation, such as the lens of the eye for neutrons.

Renogram: Plot of radioactivity measured by an external detector versus time as a radiotracer transits through the kidneys; although hippuran iodine-131 was the tracer originally used, a number of other radiopharmaceuticals may be used.

Roentgen (R): Unit of exposure for x-rays and γ-rays equivalent to 2.58×10^{-4} coulombs/kg air.

Roentgen ray: Electromagnetic radiation produced when a beam of high-speed electrons collides with a solid metal target, as in an x-ray tube; includes both characteristic x-rays and bremsstrahlung.

Roentgenogram: An image on film produced by x-rays

transmitted through the body and differentially absorbed by tissues.

Scaler: An instrument that records detected radioactivity as counts.

Scan: Term originally referring to images made of radionuclide distribution obtained with a moving detector that scanned the area of interest by moving back and forth over the area in a pattern like mowing a lawn; now refers in general to images produced by detecting radionuclide distribution.

Scanner: See Rectilinear scanner.

Scatter: Radiation traveling in a direction different from that of the primary radiation beam because of deflection by a scattering interaction.

Schilling test: Test for absorption of vitamin B_{12} done by administering radiolabeled vitamin B_{12}, giving a loading dose of nonradioactive vitamin B_{12} then measuring the radioactivity in a 24-hr urine collection; if the test is done with concomitant administration of intrinsic factor, it is called a second-stage Schilling test and is used to distinguish malabsorption attributable to intrinsic factor deficit from other causes.

Scintigraphy: The process of obtaining an image of radionuclide distribution using an Anger scintillation camera.

Scintillation camera: See Anger camera.

Scintillation counter: A detector using a solid crystal for detecting radioactivity; x-rays or γ-rays produce scintillations in the crystal as they are absorbed.

Scintillation counter, liquid: See Liquid scintillation counter.

Scintillation crystal: See Crystal, scintillation.

Scintiphoto: Photographic record from the oscilloscope of an Anger camera that depicts the distribution of radioactivity detected by the camera.

Secondary radiation: Radiation resulting from interaction of primary radiation with matter.

Selenomethionine: An analogue of the amino acid methionine in which the sulfur atom is replaced by a selenium atom.

Self-absorption: Absorption of the energy of emitted photons by the matter in which the radionuclide is located.

Semiconductor detector: Crystals of various combinations of germanium and silicon and impurities that have low conductivity properties; the creation of hole pairs by absorbed radiation permits detection of incident radiation with high resolution for energy levels.

Sensitivity: Referring to a detector, describes the ratio of detected photons to emitted photons; referring to a test, describes the ability of the test to detect a disease as the ratio of true-positive results compared with all tested with the disease.

Septa: The walls of high-density material of a collimator that define the field of view of the detector with the collimator in place.

Shielding: Material used to absorb incident radiation for purposes of radiation protection or for decreasing instrument background readings.

Shunt study: Study using a radionuclide to detect abnormal shunting of blood in the circulation, either from the left (systemic) side of the circulation to the right (pulmonary) side of the circulation or from right to left; also refers to study of a shunt placed surgically in order to divert body fluids.

Sievert (SV): SI unit of radiation dose equivalent. 1 SV = 100 rem.

Single-photon emission computed tomography: See SPECT.

Specificity: Referring to a test measures the ability of the test to exclude disease when it is absent; expressed as the ratio of true-negative results compared with all tested without the disease.

SPECT (single-photon emission computed tomography): Technique that uses a computer to reconstruct in a variety of planes (transaxial, coronal, sagittal) the distribution of a γ-emitting radionuclide detected by a scintillation camera.

Spectrometer: Instrument used to measure or sort electromagnetic radiation according to energy; see Analyzer.

Standard: A radioactive source made to simulate administered dose; used for comparison purposes to determine organ function or radionuclide distribution; also a series of radioactive sources used to calibrate detectors.

Standard deviation: The statistical variation observed in a population or series of measurements determined by the population distribution.

Static image: An image recorded when the radiopharmaceutical distribution is relatively unchanging, used to define functional organ anatomy rather than a rapidly changing process.

Statistical fluctuations: Variation in count rate caused by probabilistic nature of radioactive decay.

Statistics: See Counting statistics.

Subtraction image: An image produced by adding a reversed baseline mask to a positive image, usually with contrast media injected, to bring out the differences between the images, for example, the contrast media distribution.

T_3: Triiodothyronine, active peripheral thyroid hormone containing three iodine atoms per molecule.

T_4: Thyroxine, or tetraiodothyronine, major thyroid hormone containing four iodine atoms per molecule deiodinated to be the more active T_3 form in the periphery.

Tagged compound: See Radiopharmaceutical.

TBG: Thyroxine-binding globulin, the serum protein that carries T_4.

Technetium: Metallic element number 43, which does not exist in nature; widely used as a label in nuclear medicine in the metastable form, technetium-99m, which decays with a 6-hr half-life with the emission of a monoenergetic 140-keV γ-ray.

Thyroid-stimulating hormone: See TSH.

Thyroid uptake study (RAIU, radioactive iodine uptake): Measurement of percentage of administered iodine taken up in the thyroid gland at a particular time interval.

Thyrotropin: See TSH.

Thyrotropin-releasing hormone: See TRH.

Tomography: A means for recording image information from a selected plane or section of the body; a variety of means may be used to accept information selectively from one plane or section; images may be made directly by physical motion of target detector relative to or by computer reconstruction techniques or by a combination; see also ECT and PET.

Total-body dose: Average radiation dose to the entire body obtained by averaging the dose to different tissues and organs.

Tracer: An element or compound used to trace the handling and distribution of the same substance from which it differs physically but not chemically. It should be readily detected and should not affect the process it is used to measure. Referred to as *radiotracer* when radioactivity is the physical distinguishing feature.

Transferrin: Serum β-globulin-carrying metals, iron, indium, and gallium.

Transmission scan: Detection of radiation transmitted through the body from a source on one side of the body to the detector on the opposite side, which provides an image of body absorption densities much like a radiograph but generally lacking the detailed resolution.

TRH (thyrotropin-releasing hormone): A hypothalamic hormone governing release of TSH from the anterior pituitary.

Triolein fat absorption test: Use of iodine-131-labeled oleic acid to measure absorption of triglycerides; requires stool collection to measure excreted activity.

Tripalmitin fat utilization study: Procedure using carbon-14-labeled tripalmitin at the C-1 position to measure absorption and hepatic metabolism of tripalmitin to CO_2 and H_2O; requires CO_2 collection from breath.

TSH (thyrotropin hormone or thyroid-stimulating hormone): Hormone released from the anterior pituitary thyrotrope cells under thyroid hormone servomechanism and under influence of TRH; stimulates physiologic activity of the thyroid by activating cyclic adenosine monophosphate (cyclic AMP).

Uptake study: See Thyroid uptake study.

Venogram (radionuclide): Delineation of a portion of the venous system after downstream injection of a radiopharmaceutical.

$\dot{V}/\dot{Q}$ scan (V/P scan): A radionuclide study that provides an image measuring regional ventilation ($\dot{V}$) and an image measuring regional perfusion ($\dot{Q}$) in an attempt to correlate regional ventilation and perfusion.

Vitamin B_{12} absorption test: See Schilling test.

Wavelength (λ): Distance between corresponding points on two consecutive wavefronts; for electromagnetic radiation such as x-rays and γ-rays, it is inversely proportional to the corresponding energy of the radiation.

White blood cell study (labeled): Procedure using indium-111 oxine-labeled polymorphonuclear leukocytes to track their accumulation and thereby identify sites of pyogenic infection.

Window width: Setting of energy ranges that will be accepted by a detector; see Pulse-height analyzer.

x-Ray: A photon of electromagnetic radiation produced when an electron falls from an outer atomic orbit to fill an inner orbital vacancy created by energetic displacement of the inner orbital electron. The released photon energy is exactly the difference between the binding energies of the two shells (characteristic radiation). A spectrum of x-rays may also be produced by interaction of high energy electrons with the nucleus (bremsstrahlung radiation); see Roentgen ray.

Index

Abscess
  cerebral, 130
  hepatic, 149
  intra-abdominal, 151
Absorptiometry
  dual-photon, 185, 186
  single-photon, 185–186
Acid phosphatase, 169
Acquired immunodeficiency
      syndrome, gallium scan
      for, 151–152
ACTH
  -dependent hyperplasia, 48
  ectopic production of, 47
  -induced adrenal hyperplasia,
      48
  secretion, 47, 48
Activity, flip-flop, 128
Acute tubular necrosis (ATN),
      post-transplantation, 109
Adenocarcinoma
  bowel, 168
  breast, 167
Adenoma
  parathyroid, localization of,
      45–46
  pituitary, 49f
Adrenal cortical hyperplasia,
      49f
  bilateral, 48
Adrenal cortical uptake and
      imaging, 47–49f
Adrenal hormones, cortical syn-
      thesis of, 47
Adrenal medullary imaging, 49–
      50
Adriamycin, cardiac toxicity, 57

Aerosol studies, in pulmonary
      embolism and infarction,
      73
Aggregated albumin, 69, 203
AIDS, See Acquired im-
      munodeficiency syndrome
Air travel, radiation exposure
      from, 6
Albumin, aggregated micro-
      spheres, 69
Alcoholic liver disease, 96
Aldosterone, hypersecretion of,
      47
Alkaline phosphatase, 169
Alpha (α) particles, 3, 4
  emitters, 166
  penetration of matter, 4
Alzheimer's disease, 124
Americium-241, 187
Amines, ^{123}I-labeled, 127
Amino acids, ^{11}C-labeled, 124
p-Aminohippurate (PAH), 104
Ammonia, N-labeled, 12, 63
Anastomosis, surgical, 99
Anemia, pernicious, 179
Anger scintillation camera, 15–
      16
Angiogram
  pulmonary, for embolism,
      73
  radionuclide, 58–59, 118
    bone, 116
    cerebral, See Cerebral an-
        giography
    of liver, 140
    for spleen rupture, 141
    for spleen trauma, 140

for subdural hematoma, 139, 140
Ankylosing spondylitis, 8–9
Annihilation radiation, 17
Antigen
  concentration, increasing of, 176
  free, 176
Antigen–antibody complex, 176
Antigen–antibody reaction, specificity of, 176
Antitumor antibodies, radiolabeled, 164
APUD neoplasms, 49
Arrhythmias, cardiac, 54
Arthritis, 118, 119, 120
  septic, 120
Aspiration studies, pulmonary, 88–89
Atoms, background radiation from, 5
Attenuation
  changes, 17–18
  coefficient, 185
Autonomous nodule thyroid, 40
Autoradiographic studies, of Meckel's diverticulum, 90

Background radiation, 5–6
Bacterial overgrowth, 180
Barrett's esophagus, 90
Battered children, evaluation for bone trauma, 144
Bayes' theorem, 25
  graphic solution to, 28–29
Beta (β) particles, 3, 4
  emitters, 166
  penetration of matter, 4
Beta (β) rays, dose level and distribution, 4
Bile acid breath test, 193
Bile reflux scintigraphy, 89
Biliary fistula, 100
Biliary leakage, 99, 100

postoperative, 99
Biliary tract, 95
  biliary leakage, 99, 100
  cholecystitis, 95–98
  cholestasis, 99
  imaging, 13t
  postoperative evaluation, 99–100
  trauma, 100
Biliary tree, visualization, 95
Biopsy, liver, trauma from, 140
Bladder
  reflux, ureteral, 108
  voiding volume, renal, 108
Blind loop syndrome, 193
Blood-barrier, brain scan, 130
Blood flow, bone, 112
Blood-pool images, 118
  cardiac, 53–57
  of venous occlusive disease, 80–81
Blood volume
  defined, 181
  determination, 181–183
Body, radioactivity, 5–6
Body spaces, measurement of, 180–181, 183
  blood volume, 181–183
Bone
  blood flow, 112
  densitometry, 184
  formation and resorption, 112
  heterotopic, 121
  hyperemia, 114
  infarcts, 117
  infection, indium-111-labeled leukocytes for, 153, 154
  metabolic disease, 118
  mineral content, measurement of, 184–186
  scanning, See Bone imaging, scanning
  trauma, 142–145
  tumors, 8

turnover rates, 112
Bone imaging, scanning, 13t, 144
  abnormal, causes of, 167
  in bowel adenocarcinoma, 168
  gallium for, 155
  indium-111-labeled leukocytes for, 155
  of infection, 117–118
  for inflammatory and infectious processes, 148–149
  of metastatic disease, 118
  of neoplasms, 113–116f
  radionuclide, principles of, 112–113
  of trauma, 116–117
  of vascular disease, 117–118
Bone marrow
  imaging, 13t, 83, 121
  processes infiltrating and replacing, 114
  radiation dose, 113
Bowel, adenocarcinoma, 168
Brain
  abscess, 130
  death, 128–130
  herpes encephalitis, 130
  inflammatory and infectious processes, 130, 150
  infarct, 129f, 130
  PET imaging, 123–125
  scan, 14t, 123
    images, delayed, 130–131
    SPECT imaging, 126–127
    radionuclide, 150
  trauma, 139–140
Breast cancer
  adenocarcinoma, 167
  bone scanning in, 114
  lymphoscintigraphy for, 159–160
Breath tests, 91, 193
Bronchial
  obstruction, 71, 192
  tree, 145

Bronchogenic carcinoma, 162
  non-oat cell, 167–168
Burn victims, 145

Camera, scintillation, Anger, 15–16
Cancer, 157
  chest evaluation, 161–164
  radiation-induced, 8–9
  radioimmunodetection and radioimmunotherapy, 164–166
  radionuclide liver imaging, 157–159
  radionuclide lymphoscintigraphy, 159–161
  specific tumor types, 167–169
Capillaries, embolization of, 69
Carbon (^{11}C), positron-emitting radionuclides of, 12
Carbon-14, 5
Carcinoembryonic antigen (CEA), 164
Carcinogenesis, radiation, 8–9
Carcinoma, See specific type; specific body area
Cardiac cycle, images, 53–54
Cardiomyopathy, idiopathic, 61
Cardiopulmonary disease, nuclear medicine tests, sensitivities and specificities of, 191–192
Cardiovascular system, 53
  angiography, radionuclide, 58–59
  cardiac blood-pool imaging and evaluation of ventricular function, 53–57
  myocardial infarct imaging, 64–66
  myocardial perfusion evaluation, 59–63
  PET imaging of blood flow and metabolism, 63–64

Carfentinil, 124
Catheterization, ureteral, 103
Cathode-ray tube (CRT), 15–16
Cellular processing, radiopharmaceutical labeling customized to, 13t
Cellulitis, 118, 149
Central nervous system, 123
cerebrospinal fluid dynamics, 132–135
delayed brain scan images, 130–131
disease, nuclear medicine tests, sensitivity and specificity of, 200
PET imaging, 123–125
radionuclide cerebral angiography, 127–130
SPECT imaging, 126–127
Central nervous system (CNS) syndrome, death from, 7
Cerebral angiography, radionuclide
of cerebral death, 128, 130
of vascular problems, 127–128, 129f
Cerebral death, 128, 130
Cerebrospinal fluid
dynamics, radionuclide cisternography, 132–135
leaks, 134
Cerebrovascular accident (CVA), 128, 129f
Charcoal, 176
Chemotherapeutic agents, cardiotoxic effects, monitoring of, 164
Chemotherapy, 114
Chest
evaluation, for cancer, 161–164
roentgenograms, 151
Children
battered, 144
leukemia in, 9

use of gallium in, 153
Cholangiography, percutaneous, 100
Cholecystitis
acute, 95, 96–97
chronic, 97–98
Cholecystogram, oral, of cholecystitis, chronic, 97
Cholecystokinin (CCK), 89, 96
Cholescintigram
of cholecystitis
acute, 96–97, 98f
chronic, 97, 98
^{99m}Tc IDA, 95
for trauma, abdominal, 100
Cholestasis, 99
Cholesterol, 47
Cholinergic sites, visualization, 124
Chromosomal changes, 7
Chronic obstructive pulmonary disease, 71–76
Chylomicrons, 47
Cinematic cardiac blood-pool images, 54
Cisternography, radionuclide, 132–133
CSF leaks and shunts, 134
normal-pressure hydrocephalus, 133–134
radiopharmaceuticals for, 134–135
Coincidence counting, 17
Collateral coronary vessels, 61
Collimation, problems, 17
Collimator, 16
resolution limitations, 85
Color-coded subtraction, 45
Columnar epithelium, 90
Common duct, visualization, 97
Computed tomography (CT), 16, 17
for abdominal trauma, 140n
brain imaging, 123
of cholestasis, 99

of liver, 87
    cancer, 158
    mediastinal scans, 163, 164
Computer
    controlled subtraction, 45
    gallium uptake and, 152
Conn's syndrome of
        hyperaldosteronism, 48
Coronary artery disease, 57
Coronary artery stenosis, 60, 61
Corticosteroids, systemic, 131
Cosmic radiation, 5
Creatinine clearance, 103
^{51}Cr sodium chromate, 182
Crystal
    gamma camera, 15
    sodium iodide [NaI(Tl)], 15
Cushing's disease, 48, 49
Cyclotrons, 12
Cystic duct
    patency versus obstruction of,
        95, 96
    remnants, 99
Cystoscopy, 103

Death
    cerebral, 128, 130
    mode of, after whole body ex-
        posure, 7
Deep-vein thrombosis, 77, 78
Delayed images, 118
Diagnostic process; See also
        Tests
    predictive value, prevalence
        and Bayes' theorem, 24–
        30
Diagnostic radiation
    background level, 6
    use of, 10–11
Diastole, 53
Diphosphonate compounds, 113
Disease prevalence, effect on
        positive predictive value
        of test, 26–27
Diverticulum, Meckel's, 90–91

Dopaminergic sites, visualiza-
        tion, 124
Dose equivalent, 4
    radiation, absorbed, 3
Doubling dose, 9
Duodenum, visualization, 99
Dye dilution curves, 58

Ectopic gastric mucosa, 90
Effective renal plasma flow
        (ERPF), 104
Ejection fraction
    left ventricular, 54, 57
    right ventricular, 57
Electrocardiogram (ECG), sig-
        nals, 53
Electron, positive, 17
Embolism, pulmonary, See Pul-
        monary embolism
Encephalitis, 130
    herpes simplex, 130
End-diastolic counts (EDC), 54
End-systolic counts (ESC), 54
Endocrinologic disease, nuclear
        medicine tests, sensitivities
        and specificities of, 195–
        196
Endocrinology
    adrenal cortical uptake and
        imaging, 47–49
    adrenal medullary imaging,
        49–50
    parathyroid imaging, 44–47
    radioiodine therapy, 42–43
    thyroid carcinoma, 43
    thyroid uptake and imaging,
        35–42
Endoscopy, for gastroesophageal
        reflux, 88
Energy level, 15
Environment, radiation level in,
        4
Epididymitis, torsion versus, 110
Esophageal transit studies,
        scintigraphic, 87–88

Exercise testing
  cardiac blood-pool images in, 57
  of myocardial perfusion, 63
  thallium, 27–28
  thallium-201 chloride images in, 60
External-beam therapy, 4

False-negative (FN) results, 22
  in bone scans, 150
  in ventilation abnormalities, 53
False-positive results, 25
  receiver operating characteristic curve, 23–24
  in spleen angiography, 141
Fatigue fractures, 116–117
Fatty acids, in myocardial ischemia, 64
Feet, dorsum, radiocolloid injection in, 161
Femoral vein, left, occlusion of, 78f
Fetus, radiation exposure to, 11
Fever of unknown origin, 153
Fibrinogen uptake test, 79
Film, resolution limitations, 85
First-pass cardiac study, 58
Fistula, biliary, 100
Flip-flop, 128
Fluorescence imaging, x-ray, 12–13, 187
Fluorine-18 (^{18}F), 12
Fluoroudeoxyglucose, fluorine-18-labeled (^{18}F FDG), 64
  PET brain image, 124, 125f
Fracture
  bone, 116–117
    hairline, 143
    stress, 142, 144f
  kidney, 140
  rib, 142
  spleen, 140

Gallbladder
  filling, 97
  nonvisualization of, 97, 98f
  visualization of, 89
    delayed, 98
Gallium-67 (^{67}Ga) citrate, 164
  bone scan with, 118
  for inflammatory and infectious processes, 150–153, 154, 155
  mediastinal scan, 162–163, 163f
Gallium-68 (^{68}Ga), 12–13, 18
Gallium scan
  for bronchogenic carcinoma, 168
  of hepatic cancer, 158
  liver–spleen, 148–149
  for lung cancer, 162
  of osteomyelitis, 150
Gamma camera, scintillation crystal, 15
Gamma (γ) emitting radionuclide, 11
Gamma (γ) rays, 3, 4
  detection of, 15
  direction of travel, 16
  dose level and distribution, 4
  energy distribution, 4
  measured exposure level, 4
  scintillation imaging, 7
Gastric emptying, 89
Gastric mucosa
  ectopic, 90
  uptake, 13t
Gastroesophageal reflux, 88
Gastrointestinal disease, nuclear medicine tests, sensitivity and specificity of, 192–193
Gastrointestinal function tests, 91
Gastrointestinal hemorrhage, acute, 91–92
Gated cardiac imaging, 53–57

Geiger counter, 4
Genetic effects of radiation, 6,
      9–11
Genetically significant dose
      (GSD), 10
Genitourinary disease, nuclear
      medicine tests, sensitivity
      and specificity of, 198–
      199
Genitourinary tract, 102
   hydronephrosis or possible
      obstruction, 105–108
   renal function evaluation,
      103–104
   renal parenchymal masses,
      108–109
   renal transplantation, 109
   renovascular hypertension,
      109
   scrotal imaging, 110
   ureteral reflux, 108
Glomerular filtration rate
      (GFR), measurement, 104
Glossary, 203–225
Glucocorticoid synthesis, 47
Glucoheptonate, for renal
      parenchymal masses, 108–
      109
Glucose, cerebral utilization,
      125f
Goiters, 39
   toxic, 41
Graves' disease, 41, 42
Gray (Gy), 3, 4
Growth stimulating antibodies,
      39
Gy (Gray), 4

Hairline fractures, 143
Half-life, 213
Hands, dorsum, radiocolloid in-
      jection in, 161
Hashimoto's thyroiditis, 42
Head, trauma, 139–140
Heart, scan, 164
Hematocrit, 182

   decreased, 182
   measured, dependence on,
      182–183
   whole-body, 182
Hematologic disorders, nuclear
      medicine tests, sensitivity
      and specificity, 197
Hematoma
   intrahepatic, 140
   spleen, 140
   subdural, 139–140
Hematopoietic syndromes
   death from, 7
   treatment, 7
Hemorrhage, gastrointestinal,
      acute, 91–92
Hepatobiliary study, normal, 96f
Hepatocellular disease, 83, 85f
Hepatocyte, imaging, 13t
HIDA for hepatocyte imaging,
      89, 95, 141, 213
Hip(s), aseptic necrosis, 117
Hippuran, 105, 106f
   excretion, 104
Hiroshima survivors, 8, 9
Hirsutism, 48
Human immunodeficiency virus
      (HIV), 152
Huntington's disease, 124
Hybridoma technology, 165
Hydrocephalus, normal-
      pressure, 133f, 133–134
Hydronephrosis, 105–108
Hyperaldosteronism, Conn's
      syndrome of, 48
Hyperbaric technique, for
      radiopharmaceutical ad-
      ministration, 132
Hypercorticalism, 48
Hyperemia, 128
Hyperparathyroidism, primary,
      45
Hypertension
   pulmonary, 69
   renovascular, 109
Hyperthyroidism, 41

of Graves' disease, therapy, 42
toxic goiters causing, 41
Hypothyroidism
  congenital, sporadic, 40
  in Graves' disease, therapy, 42

Ileum, Meckel's diverticulum in,
  90–91
Iliopelvic lymphoscintigraphy,
  161
Images, formation of, 3
Imaging, of radiation, 15–16
Iminodiacetic acid (IDA) com-
  pounds, 89
Immunoglobulin G (IgG), 176
Indium-111 (^{111} In), for cancer
  therapy, 166
Indium-111 DTPA cisternogram
  images, 133f, 134
Indium-111-labeled antibody
  imaging, 165, 166f
Indium-111-labeled leukocytes
  for inflammatory and in-
    fectious processes, 151,
    153f, 153–155
  for liver–spleen scan, 149
Indium-111 platelets, 81
Infection, bone, 117–118
Infectious disease, nuclear medicine tests, sensitivity and
  specificity of, 196–197
Infectious processes, See Inflammatory and infectious
  processes
Inflammatory and infectious
  processes
  imaging of, 14t, 148
  gallium-67 imaging, 150–153
  indium-111-labeled leukocytes,
    153–155
  multiorgan imaging, 148–150
Internal mammary lymph
  nodes, in breast carcinoma, 167
Internal mammary lymphoscintigraphy, 159–160

Interstitial lung disease, 70
Intra-abdominal infection, 151
  indium-111-labeled leukocytes
    imaging for, 153–154
Intradermal lymphoscintigraphy, 160–161
Iodide
  deficiency, 39
  oxidation of, 35
Iodide pool, expansion of, 36
Iodine
  determination, 187
  radioactive, 7
  uptake, 35–36
Iodine-123 (^{123}I), 19, 35, 165
  thyroid imaging with, 38, 39
  discordant changes in, 39
Iodine-123-labeled amines, 127
Iodine-123-labeled hippuran,
  127
  for renal function studies,
    104
Iodine-123-labeled iodoamphetamine (^{123}IMP), 127
Iodine-125 (^{125}I) fibrinogen uptake test, for lower-
  extremity deep vein
  thrombosis, 79–80
Iodine-125 iothalamate, glomerular filtration rate detection with, 104
Iodine-125-labeled human
  serum albumin, 182
Iodine-131(^{131}I), 9, 164, 166
  thyroid imaging with, 38
  for carcinoma, 43
Iodine-131 hippuran (OIH)
  activity, 107f, 107
  for renal function studies,
    103–104
Iodine-131-labeled metabenzyl-
  guaninidine (MIBG),
  adrenal medullary imag-
  ing with, 49–50
Iodine-131-labeled norcholesterol, 47–48

Iodine-131 orthiodohippurate (hippuran), 141–142
Iodoantipyrine, 183
Iodothyronines, 35
Iodotyrosines, 35
Ionization, 4
Ionization chamber, 4
Ionizing radiation, forms of, 3
Iron, 183
Ischemia, 114
Ischemic brain disease, 127, 128
Ischemic heart disease, 57
Isotope dilution, 180–181, 182

Jaundice, obstructive, 99
Joint disease, 118, 119
    nuclear medicine tests, sensitivity and specificity of, 194

Kaposi's sarcoma, 152
Kidney
    function, *See* Renal function
    trauma, 141–142
Knee, meniscal tears, 144–145
Krypton-81m (^{81m}Kr), 70

Lactic acidosis, 128
Laminar cortical necrosis, 130
Lead-210, 6
Leukemia, 8, 9
    from ^{131}I therapy, 43
    incidence of, 7
Ligand binding, competitive, 176
Linear effect, 9, 9n
Lipoproteins, low-density, 47
Liver
    abnormalities, focal, 85–86
    cancer, radionuclide imaging, 157–159
    disease, nuclear medicine tests, sensitivity and specificity of, 193–194
    imaging, 13t

metastases, 83
    from bowel adenocarcinoma, 168
    from bronchogenic carcinoma, 168
    scanning, in prostate cancer, 169
    trauma, 140
    tumors, 83
Liver–spleen imaging, 83–87
    for inflammatory and infectious processes, 148–149
Lobulations, 140
Lower extremities, venous system, visualization, 76–78
Lung
    biological half-life of lung scanning particles, 69
    cancer, 8, 161–162
        staging, 163
    embolic disease, 73
    infarcted, 73
    interstitial disease, 70
    scan, 13t
        interpretation, 70
        for pulmonary embolism, 68
    trauma, 145
Lymph channels, visualization of, 159
Lymph nodes, visualization of, 159
Lymphoscintigraphy, radionuclide, 159–161

Macroaggregated albumin, 69, 76
Magnetic resonance imaging (MRI), 3, 16, 17
    brain imaging, 123
    for meniscal tears in knee, 144–145
    for subdural hematoma, 139
Malignant melanoma, lymphatic drainage from, 160

Meckel's diverticulum, 90–91
Mediastinoscopies, 163
Mediastinum
  imaging over, 40
  scan, 90–91
  upper, images, 45
Meningitis, 130
Meniscal tears, 144–145
Metabolic disease, of bone, 118
Metabolic function, determination, 183
Millirad, 3
Mineral, bone content, 184–186
Monoclonal antibodies
  labeled, 164
  tumor imaging with, 165
Morison's pouch, 148
Morphine for biliary tract imaging, 96
Morphologic images, 17
MRI, *See* Magnetic resonance imaging
MUGA study, 53
Muscle disease, nuclear medicine tests, sensitivity and specificity of, 194–195
Myocardial blood flow and metabolism, PET imaging of, 63–64, 64f
Myocardial infarction, 60
  imaging, 64, 65–66
Myocardial ischemia, 60
  PET images of, 64
  stress-induced, 57
Myocardial perfusion
  evaluation, 59–63
  imaging, 13t

N-isopropyl, 127
Nagasaki survivors, 8, 9
Natural radiation, 5–6
Natural risk, doubling of, 9
Neck
  images, 45
  vessels, 127

Neoplasms, *See* Tumors
Neuroreceptors, PET imaging of, 124
Neutron, 4
Nitrogen (^{13}N), positron-emitting radionuclides of, 12
Nodules, thyroid, 39–40
  autonomous, 40
  nonfunctioning (cold), 41–42
Nonimaging procedures, 175
  measuring body spaces, 180–183
  quantitative tests, 184–187
  radioligand assays, 175–178
  Schilling test, 178–180
Non-oat cell bronchogenic carcinoma, 167–168
Norcholesterol ^{131}I-labeled, 47–48
Normal distribution of test results, 212
NP-59, 47
Nuclear weapons, radiation associated with, 4

Obstructive pulmonary disease, 71
Opiate receptors, visualization, 124
Opportunistic infections, 151
Ossification, ectopic, 121
Osteomyelitis, 117–118, 149–150
  gallium imaging for, 152–153
Osteoarthropathy, 194
Osteogenic sarcoma, 162
Osteoporosis, 118
  nuclear medicine tests, sensitivity and specificity of, 195
Osteoporotic process, 185
Ovaries, ectopic thyroid tissue in, 41
Oxygen (^{15}O), positron-emitting radionuclides of, 12

Paget's disease, 114, 116f, 118
Pancreatic enzyme, lack of, 180
Pancreatitis, 96
Paraganglionoma, 49
Parathyroid imaging, 44–47
Parenchyma
  pulmonary
    disease, 73
    neoplasm, 168
  renal
    masses, 108–109
    processes, 149
Pedal veins, radiopharmaceutical
    injection into, 77
Pelvimetry, 9
Pelvis, imaging of, 142
Peptic ulcer disease, 88, 89
Perchlorate washout test, 37
Perfusion imaging, pulmonary,
    69–70, 71
  for nonembolic pulmonary
    disease, 76
  for pulmonary embolism, 68
Pernicious anemia, 179
Periosteal injuries, 142, 143
Pertechnetate (TcO$_4$), 12; See
    also Technetium-99m per-
    technetate
  for ectopic thyroid tissue, 40
PET, See Positron emission
    tomography
Pheochromocytomas, adrenal,
    49, 50, 50f
Phosphonate compounds,
    ^{99m}Tc-complexed, 113
Photomultiplier tube, 15
Physiologic function, evaluation
    of, 175
Pinhole collimator, 16
Plasma, volume, 181, 182
Platelets, ^{111}In, 81
Pneumocystis carinii, 152
Polonium-210, 6
Polyclonal antibodies,
    radiolabeled, 164–165

Polyphosphate, 113
Portal hypertension, 83
Positron(s), 17
Positron detector, 17
Positron emission tomography
    (PET)
  of brain, 123–125
  features, 16–18
  of myocardial blood flow and
    metabolism, 63–64, 64f
Positron-emitting radionuclides,
    18
Potassium, radioactive, 5, 183
Predictive value, of tests, posi-
    tive, 25–27
Pregnancy, radiation exposure
    in, 11
Probability, prior, 24
Process rates, disturbance in, 30
Prostate cancer
  bone scan in, 115f
  metastases, 168–169
Pulmonary aspiration studies,
    88–89
Pulmonary disease, nonembolic,
    76
Pulmonary embolism
  detection of, pulmonary per-
    fusion sensitivity in, 71
  diagnosis, 68
  specificity of radionuclide pul-
    monary perfusion imag-
    ing, 71–76
Pulmonary hypertension, 69
Pulmonary infection, gallium
    imaging of, 151
Pulmonary parenchyma, See
    Parenchyma, pulmonary
Pulmonary perfusion/ventilation
    imaging, 70
  principles, 69–70
  in pulmonary embolism,
    sensitivity and specificity
    of, 71–76
Pulmonary vascular disease, 73

Pyelography, 103
Pyrophosphate, 113

Quantity exposure, 4
Quinuclidinyl benzilate (QNB), 124

Rad, 3, 4
  dose of, 3–4
Radiation; See also specific type
  bone changes from, 114
  carcinogenesis, 8–9
  defined, 3
  dose, 3
    specification of, 3–4
  effects, 6–11
  high-level doses, somatic
    effects, 6–8
  imaging of, 15–16
  nonionizing, 3
  risks from, 6
Radiation detection devices, 4
Radiation necrosis, 131
Radiation therapy, effects, 131
Radioactivity, natural, 5
Radiofrequency (RF), 3
  signal, 3
Radioimmunoassay (RIA), 175
Radioiodide, 7–8
Radioiodine therapy, 42–43
Radioisotope, 219
Radioligand assays (RIA), 175–177
  clinical uses, 177–178
Radiopharmaceuticals, 11–13
  labeling, customized to cellular
    lar processes, 13t
  perfusion, decreased, focal regions of, 128
  positron-labeled, 18
  for renal function studies, 103–104
Radon, 8
Rb, See Rubidium

Receiver operating characteristic
  (ROC) curve, 23–24
Red cell; See also Technetium-
  99m red blood cells
  mass, 181–182
Reflux
  bile, 89
  gastroesophageal, 88
  ureteral, 108
Renal column of Bertin, 109
Renal function, evaluation of, 14t, 103
  radiopharmaceuticals for, 103–104
Renal imaging, 14t
Renal scintigraphy, 149
  information obtained from, 102
Renal transplantation, 109
Renogram, diuretic-augmented, 107
Renovascular hypertension, 109
Resolution, limitations, 85
Rhabdomyolysis, 121, 195
Rheumatoid arthritis, 113, 118, 194
Rib, fractures, 142
Right ventricular hypertrophy, 61,
Roentgen (R), 4
Rubidium-82 (^{82}Rb), 18, 63
  generator systems producing, 12

Schilling test, 26, 175, 178–180
Scintigraphy
  for bile duct obstruction, 99
  bile reflux, 89
  gastroesophageal, 88
  renal, 102, 149
Scintillation camera
  Anger, 15–16
  resolution limitations, 85
Scintillation counter, liquid, 214

Scrotal imaging, 110
Semiconductor detectors, 222
Sensitivity, of nuclear medicine
        tests, 21, 22–23, 191–201
Serum resin T3 uptake test, 177
Shin splints, 227
Shunt
   lesions, 58–59
   patency, 134
Sialitis, 7
   radiation, 43
Sickle cell disease, 117
Single-photon emission com-
        puted tomography
        (SPECT)
   of brain, 126–127
   features, 18–19
   of hepatic cancer, 158
   mediastinal, 163
   of meningeal tears in knee,
        144–145
   of myocardial infarction, 66
   of myocardial perfusion, 60,
        63
   of spondylolysis, 145
Skeletal system
   bone, See Bone
   joint disease, 118–120
   nuclear medicine tests,
        sensitivity and specificity
        of, 194
   soft tissue lesions, 120–121
Sodium, radioactive, 183
Sodium/potassium ATPase
        pump, 44, 59
Soft tissue
   infection, 118
   lesions, 120–121
Somatic changes, from high-
        level radiation doses, 6–8
x-y spatial coordinate, 15
Sonography, See Ultrasound
Specificities, of nuclear medicine
        tests, 21, 23, 191–201

SPECT, See Single-photon emis-
        sion computed tomogra-
        phy
Spermatic cord, torsion, 110
Sphincter of Oddi, 97
Spiperone, 124
Spleen; See also Liver–spleen im-
        aging
   hooked, 140
   imaging, 13t
   trauma, 140
Spondylolysis, 145
Steroid, synthesis, 48
Stomach
   distended, 140
   imaging of, 89
Stress fracture, 116–117, 141,
        144f
Struma ovarii, 41
Subdural hematoma (SDH),
        139–140
Subtraction
   color-coded, 45
   computer-controlled, 45
Surgery
   for parathyroid adenoma, 44–
        47
   for thyroid disease, 28
Survival time, after whole-body
        exposure, 7
Systole, 53

T3, See Triiodothyronine
T4, See Thyroxine
T-tube study, 100
99mTc, See Technetium-99m
Technetium-99m (99mTc), 11–
        12, 19, 165
   bone scan, 153
   distributions, 45
   liver–spleen scan, 149
   particle injection, for throm-
        bus detection, 77f
   radiopharmaceuticals, 13–14t

thyroid imaging with, 39
for ureteral reflux, 108
Technetium-99m (^{99m}Tc) antimony trisulfide colloid,
for lymphoscintigraphy, 159, 160f
Technetium-99m (^{99m}Tc) colloid
for bone marrow scan, 117, 121
for liver trauma, 140
for spleen trauma, 140
Technetium-99m (^{99m}Tc) complex, for renal function studies, 103
Technetium-99m (^{99m}Tc)-complexed phosphonate compounds, 113
Technetium-99m (^{99m}Tc) diethylenetriaminepentaacetic acid (DTPA), 12, 141, 149
for cisternography, 134, 135
for hydronephrosis or obstruction, 108
for renal function studies, 104
for thrombus detection, 78
ventilation imaging with, 70
Technetium-99m (^{99m}Tc) dimercaptosuccinic acid (DMSA), 141, 149
for renal function study, 104
for renal parenchymal masses, 108–109
Technetium-99m (^{99m}Tc) diphosphonate, 113
bone imaging, for lung cancer, 162
Technetium-99m (^{99m}Tc)-dl-hexamethylpropyleneamine oximine (HMPAO), 126–127
Technetium-99m (^{99m}Tc) glucoheptonate, 129f, 131f, 141, 149

for hydronephrosis or obstruction, 105, 105f
for renal function studies, 104
Technetium-99m (^{99m}Tc) iminodiacetic acid (IDA)
for biliary leakage, 99
for biliary tree visualization, 95, 96f
for cholestasis, 99
acute, 96–97, 98f
chronic, 97, 98
hepatobiliary imaging, for postoperative evaluation, 99–100
for liver trauma, 140
Technetium-99m (^{99m}Tc) iron ascorbate DTPA, for renal function study, 104
Technetium-99m (^{99m}Tc) isonitrile compounds, for myocardial perfusion, 62, 62f, 63
Technetium-99m (^{99m}Tc)-labeled agents, for vascular disease, 142
Technetium-99m (^{99m}Tc)-labeled to albumin macroaggregates
for pulmonary perfusion imaging, 69, 72
for thrombus detection, 76
Technetium 99-m (^{99m}Tc)-labeled to albumin microspheres, for pulmonary perfusion imaging, 69
Technetium-99m (^{99m}Tc)-labeled phosphate
bone scanning with, 117, 144, 149
for soft tissue lesions, 120–121
Technetium-99m (^{99m}Tc) MDP, bone scan, 115f, 153f

Technetium-99m (^{99m}Tc) mercaptoacetyltriglycine (MAG$_3$), for renal function studies, 104
Technetium-99m (^{99m}Tc) pertechnetate
  for ectopic gastric mucosa, 90
  free, 92
  for Meckel's diverticulum, 90–91
  for scrotal imaging, 110
  thyroid imaging with, 38f, 38
    discordant images in, 39
  uptake, in neck regions, 44
Technetium-99m (^{99m}Tc) pyrophosphate, myocardial infarct imaging with, 64–66
Technetium-99m (^{99m}Tc) red blood cells, 53
  for acute gastrointestinal hemorrhage, 91, 92
  blood pool images of pelvis with, 80f, 81
  heat damaged, for splenic trauma, 141
  for liver imaging, 87
Technetium-99m (^{99m}Tc) sodium pertechnetate, 58
Technetium-99m (^{99m}Tc) sulfur colloid, 12
  for acute gastrointestinal hemorrhage, 91, 92
  for esophageal transit studies, 87–88
  flow to bone marrow, 83
  for gastroesophageal reflux, 88
  for hepatic cancer, 158f
  for liver–spleen scan, 83, 148, 154, 155
  for pulmonary aspiration studies, 88–89
Test
  results
    false-negative, 22; See also False-negative results
    true-positive, 22; See also True-positive results
    value, 28
  sensitivity and specificity, 21, 22–23, 191–192
Tetraiodothyronine (T4), See Thyroxine
Thallium-201 (^{201}Tl), 45
  stress test, positive, 27–28
  uptake
    myocardial, 59
    in brain tumors versus radiation necrosis, 124
    in neoplasms, 44
Thallium-201 (^{201}Tl) chloride, myocardial perfusion evaluation with, 59, 60, 61–64
Thallium-technetium pertechnetate subtraction imaging, parathyroid gland, 44–47
Therapeutic radioiodine
  for hyperthyroidism, 42
  for neuroblastoma, MIBG, 49
  for thyroid cancer, 43
Therapeutic irradiation, somatic changes from, 7
Thorax, bone scintigraphy of, 162
Thorotrast, 8
Thrombus, detection, 76–81
Thymic irradiation, 8
Thyroglobulin, 35
Thyroid cancer, 8, 9
Thyroid disease, radioiodine therapy for, 42–43
Thyroid hormone
  biosynthesis, 35
  studies, 177–178
Thyroid stimulating hormone (TSH), 39
  endogenous, 43

exogenous, 43
stimulation and suppression of, 36–37
Thyroid uptake and imaging, 35, 37–39
  of abnormalities, 41–42
  of ectopic thyroid tissue, 40–41
  perchlorate washout test, 37
  radioactive iodine, 35–36
  of thyroid nodules, 39–40
  TSH stimulation and suppression, 36–37
Thyroiditis
  acute suppurative, 42
  Hashimoto's, 42
  radiation, 43
  subacute, 42
Thyrotropin-releasing hormone (TRH), stimulation and suppression, 36–37
Thyroxine (tetraiodothyronine, T4), 35, 176, 177
  free, 35, 177
Thyroxine-binding globulin (TBG), 177, 178
Time-activity curve, 58, 59
²⁰¹Tl, See Thallium-201
Tomography, See CT, MRI, PET, SPECT
Torsion, spermatic cord, versus, epididymitis, 110
Total body dose, 10
Trabecular bone, 185, 186
Tracer
  distribution, 19
  in PET, 18
  theory in disease, 23
Transplantation, renal, 109
Trauma, 139
  abdominal, 100
  bone, 116–117, 142–145
  brain, 139–140
  kidney, 141–142
  liver, 140

lung, 145
spleen, 140–141
vascular, 142
TRH, See Thyrotropin-releasing hormone
Triglyceride, labeled, 183
Triiodothyronine (T3), 35, 176, 177
  free, 35
  uptake test, serum resin, 177
Triolein fat absorption test, 224
Tripalmitin fat absorption test, 224
True-negative results, 25
True-positive (TP) results, 22
Tumor
  antigens, 164–166
  bone, 113–116f
  brain, 124
  doubling time, 157
  imaging, 13t
    with gallium, 150–151
  nuclear medicine tests, sensitivity and specificity of, 197–198
  radioimmunoimaging, 164–166
  radioimmunotherapy, 164–166

Ultrasound, 3
  of cholecystitis, 99
    acute, 97
    chronic, 97
  of liver, 87
    cancer, 158
  of thyroid nodules, 42
Upper gastrointestinal contrast studies, for gastroesophageal reflux, 88
Upper gastrointestinal series, 100
Uptake, radioiodine for thyroid function, 35–36

Ureteral catheterization, 103
Ureteral obstruction, 105–108
Ureteral reflux, 108
Ureterovesical stone, 105
Urine
  leakage, 141
  radioactive vitamin B_{12} in,
    179–180
Urinomas, 141
Urography, 103

Vascular disease, 117
  nuclear medicine tests,
    sensitivity and specificity
    of, 201
Vascular lesions, 142
Vascular problems, brain, 127–
  128, 129f
Vasculitis, 114
Venogram
  contrast, for thrombus detec-
    tion, 78, 79
  lower extremity, thrombus,
    77, 78, 79
  radionuclide, 76
    for thrombus detection, 78,
    79
Ventilation imaging, 69–70
  for nonembolic pulmonary
    disease, 76
Ventilation/perfusion mismatch,
  71, 73, 74f

Ventricular function, evaluation,
  53–57, 58
Ventricular hypertrophy, 61
Ventricular wall motion,
  abnormalities, 53, 54, 55f,
  56, 57
Vertebra, collapsed, 143
Vitamin B_{12}
  absorption, 175
  deficiency, 178–179
  malabsorption, 179
  serum levels, measurement,
  179

Washin images, 72f
White blood cell imaging, 151
Window, *See* Energy level

Xenon-127, 70
Xenon-133 (^{133}Xe)
  for lung trauma, 144
  for nonembolic pulmonary
    disease, 76
  ventilation images, 69, 70,
    72f, 74f
x-rays, 3, 4
  bone, 112
  dose level and distribution, 4
  energy distribution, 4
  fluorescence imaging, 12–13,
    187
  measured exposure level, 4
  plain, for lung cancer, 161